PENGUIN BOOKS

LOPSIDED

Meredith Norton lives with her son in Sonoma County, California. *Lopsided* is her first book.

To access Penguin Readers Guides online,
visit our Web sites at www.penguin.com
or www.vpbookclub.com.

MEREDITH NORTON

Lopsided

PENGUIN BOOKS

PENGUIN BOOKS
Published by the Penguin Group
Penguin Group (USA) Inc., 375 Hudson Street, New York, New York 10014, U.S.A.
Penguin Group (Canada), 90 Eglinton Avenue East, Suite 700, Toronto,
Ontario, Canada M4P 2Y3 (a division of Pearson Penguin Canada Inc.)
Penguin Books Ltd, 80 Strand, London WC2R 0RL, England
Penguin Ireland, 25 St Stephen's Green, Dublin 2, Ireland
(a division of Penguin Books Ltd)
Penguin Group (Australia), 250 Camberwell Road, Camberwell,
Victoria 3124, Australia (a division of Pearson Australia Group Pty Ltd)
Penguin Books India Pvt Ltd, 11 Community Centre, Panchsheel Park,
New Delhi – 110 017, India
Penguin Group (NZ), 67 Apollo Drive, Rosedale, North Shore 0632,
New Zealand (a division of Pearson New Zealand Ltd)
Penguin Books (South Africa) (Pty) Ltd, 24 Sturdee Avenue,
Rosebank, Johannesburg 2196, South Africa

Penguin Books Ltd, Registered Offices:
80 Strand, London WC2R 0RL, England

First published in the United States of America by Viking Penguin,
a member of Penguin Group (USA) Inc. 2008
Published in Penguin Books 2009

1 3 5 7 9 10 8 6 4 2

THE LIBRARY OF CONGRESS HAS CATALOGED THE HARDCOVER EDITION AS FOLLOWS:
Norton, Meredith.
Lopsided: how having breast cancer can be really distracting / Meredith Norton.
p. cm.
ISBN 978-0-670-01928-1 (hc.)
ISBN 978-0-14-311563-2 (pbk.)
1. Norton, Meredith—Health.   2. Breast—Cancer—Patients—Biography.   I. Title.
RC280.B8N677 2007
362.196'994490092—dc22
[B]   2007040496

Printed in the United States of America
Set in ITC Esprit Book
Designed by Francesca Belanger

AUTHOR'S NOTE

My sister has called me a liar at nearly every meal we've shared since I started talking in 1972. Back then I'd pop the bottle out of my mouth, say something unbelievable, and pop the bottle back in. I am not a liar. However, I am a storyteller. (Although, a storyteller with a good lawyer changes names and identifying characteristics and details to protect herself and the privacy of her characters, as I have done.) This book is my attempt to communicate an experience as I perceived it. It is not an affidavit. Try to enjoy it for what it is worth.

for Thibault, now you will finally
know how much you meant to me
September 10, 2007

Lopsided

chapter one

Before I moved to France my medical problems were few, minor, and real. They were things like allergies, conjunctivitis due to sharing eyeliner, and a broken pinkie from slamming the car hood on my hand. Normal problems. But once I landed in Paris and became a professional girlfriend, living in the crappy suburbs, I started developing issues. Thibault, then my boyfriend and now my husband, said it was because I spent too much time on the Internet. Of course my toes were sore; it was not due to a strange new syndrome I'd developed, but because I'd been clipping and cleaning the nails maniacally since reading that Croatian kid's Web site devoted to ingrown toenails. "And," he added, "stop sending *zose* macabre pictures of his *foongal* infections to me at work, please. You know I check my personal e-mails during lunch."

In France, every couple of months I had a new problem that required a doctor's office visit. Mostly these were small issues I overreacted to, like when my nose started whistling. But some things were scary, like when in the middle of a sentence I threw a glass of water in my own face and passed out cold. When I finally opened my eyes I couldn't decide who to acknowledge first, Thibault's mother, who sat on the bed looking glamorous in that effortless way only French women can, while she worked socks onto my feet, or the four foxy paramedics staring at me with folded arms. Thibault stood nearby looking terrified until I said, pointing to the hottest medic, "Shouldn't one of you be dressing me?"

Each trip to the doctor's office or hospital involved some insult or embarrassment. The time I got a chest X-ray, the machine was set up opposite a door facing the emergency waiting room. First the tech insisted I take off my shirt and stand topless even though the whole point of an X-ray is that it can see through things. Then he refused to lock the door so all sorts of people kept opening it to look at me standing there half-naked.

Mostly the doctors eyed me suspiciously and found creative ways to discourage future visits, as if I'd flown all the way to France simply to exploit their subsidized health care system. Their tactics didn't work; I kept subjecting myself to their cruelty until I finally got married, got a work permit, and found a job. Suddenly, without the empty days to contemplate my health, the peculiar array of psychosomatic symptoms disappeared.

I didn't see another doctor until a prepregnancy consultation for vitamin supplements. True to form, the doctor told me I was absurd, that Americans were obsessed with artificial nutrition, and that folic acid wasn't necessary until the pregnancy had been confirmed. The proclamation of his negative opinion of my fellow countrymen was expected. What I did not expect was his dismissal of the two journal reports I placed before him encouraging extra folic acid intake during the two weeks immediately following conception, namely the two weeks before pregnancy confirmation. Without bothering to pick them up he said, "You are free to waste your money on whatever you want."

I hated French doctors. It wasn't just the snotty attitudes and their dingy waiting rooms; I hated their frankness, and their liberal use of Latin. Most of all, I hated that certain way they had of ensuring that potentially pleasant situations would turn out unpleasantly.

A few months later, when I scheduled the appointment to confirm my pregnancy I prepared myself for the worst: "No, the baby is dead, see it there, that little spot, but no heartbeat. *Tant pis*." But I tried to maintain an optimism that this experience would be a positive one. Sitting in the cheap armchair trying not to hear anything the obstetrician said, I took inventory of the room, counting plaques and trying to identify the parts of a dismantled plastic torso model. My eyes stopped on the examining table. Why was it there like that, just sitting in his office? Why wasn't it in an exam room or behind a curtain or something? It was not being stored temporarily; there was a roll of crinkled paper pulled across it, and a waste bin with some inside-out rubber gloves, paper towels, and a used plastic speculum in full view. This looked nothing like an American gynecologist's office where everything is discreetly nongraphic and oven mitts protect sensitive soles from cold steel stirrups, as if you might not be there to get a Pap smear, but a steaming hot casserole.

The doctor was clearly repeating his request. "Please undress so we can get to the exam."

"Huh?" My eyes stayed fixed on the jumbo jar of lubricant jelly.

"Please undress."

"Where?" I looked around for a door or closet. Maybe he was going to step out.

"Please undress and lie down on the table."

"*Où?*" I said it very slowly and sounded like a ghost, *Oooooooooooooooo.*

"Meredith, take off your clothes and lie down," said Thibault, who looked straight ahead and spoke through clenched teeth, as if by not moving his lips the doctor couldn't hear him. He had that phony smile he always wore when I embarrassed him, the one that said, "I find this amusing," when clearly he didn't. It is the smile he wore for the first three months I was exposed to his family.

"I'm supposed to take my clothes off in front of you two?"

"I am a doctor, Madame; I assure you I have seen undressed women before."

"But what about him?" I pointed to Thibault.

"He is your husband. Depending on the results of this exam, I can assume he has seen an undressed woman before as well." Then he picked his nose staring me squarely in the face.

I stood up and began to unbutton my pants right there in front of his desk. They resumed their conversation about the paperwork we needed to file before my fourteenth week of pregnancy.

"May I have a dress, please?" I practically yelled.

"A what?"

"A paper dress, or blanket, something to cover myself with."

"A paper blanket?" he asked, totally perplexed.

I lay down on the table, stark naked, while he did a pelvic

4

exam, explained to my husband the benefits of bureaucracy, and laughed about puritanical American double standards, misplaced modesty and my limited vocabulary. I cried all the way home. My usually overly empathetic husband just stared at me as if I'd started eating sand by the spoonful.

chapter two

O ne and a half humiliation-packed years later I was thirty-four with an eleven-month-old son, just shy of my two-year wedding anniversary. After years of traveling back and forth between Europe and California for a variety of reasons, mostly nonsensical, but almost always involving weather preference, Thibault and I had finally, just three months earlier, decided to stay put in Paris. The employment opportunities and proximity to the in-laws were benefits that far outweighed my fear of living under an autocratic bureaucracy so controlling that we couldn't even name our own son Chance because some random employee at the Académie thought it sounded too feminine. We packed and shipped all our stuff from apartments and parental basements around the world to a grown-up flat in the fifteenth arrondissement with swanky Hausmannian details and a concierge. We bought non-IKEA furniture, and I dug in for the first time in my adult life. Until motherhood and marriage limited me, I had never stopped indulging my whims long enough to get settled. This time, however, I was finally ready to put my own address, not my parents', on my checks.

Thibault dressed up each day in a suit and open-necked shirt and scooted off to do whatever it is consultants do. I wore suede boots, even in the snow, and shopped at the Bon Marché Épicerie, where in addition to all the French staples, they offer Bush's baked beans, imported from the United States, for only five dollars a can. We ate duck three times a week, vacationed at Thibault's parents' country house, and I listened to Johnny Hallyday while preparing lunch. My son, Lucas, and I took aimless bus rides and visited puppet shows in parks. We took pictures of ourselves in front of the Eiffel Tower and Sacré Coeur.

Living in Paris sounded romantic. My parents loved answering their friends' inquiries about me with, "Oh, Meredith is still in Paris." The fact that I was doing nothing, had no career or plans for a career was irrelevant. Were I in Oakland they'd have had to look away and change the subject, but doing nothing in Paris was bragworthy.

Exploring Paris was entertaining, but while they say it takes years to really discover the city, it actually doesn't. A few months of methodical sightseeing will exhaust all the worthwhile destinations. Then you're reduced to sewer and morgue tours, or visiting each of the locations mentioned in *The Da Vinci Code.* You find yourself supremely depressed, standing in front of Napoleon's stuffed Arabian mare. She's so old and scrawny you want to cry. Her head is resting on a crutch and her fur has fallen out in patches, exposing the taxidermist's crude stitches. She's like a cross between a horse and a baseball, and smaller than my friend's mastiff. This is the same animal you saw depicted rearing gloriously over bloody battle scenes, under angry skies, just yesterday in the Musée d'Orsay.

In reality, living in Paris wasn't romantic; it was highly stressful. Parisians are a stressed population in general, but being an American in France, a country still bristling from its demoted status as world leader, was especially taxing. Rarely a cocktail hour passed without my screaming that I didn't vote for George Bush, didn't like George Bush, and didn't want to talk about George Bush. And I simply did not know any of those 73 percent of adult Americans that couldn't spell *America*. This, at least, was a lower percentage than the 74 percent of Frenchmen who don't wash their penises each day, a statistic I'd recently learned from a British glossy and screamed at one of Thibault's biggest consulting clients.

I feared that Thibault's marrying an American worked against him professionally so I made an effort to ingratiate myself before my husband's company went bankrupt and I ended up on the street. We invited the client to our apartment for dinner.

That day I woke up early to do my shopping. I stopped at seven stores, none of which was conveniently next door to another. At some point I lost one of the wheels on my caddy and ended up dragging the groceries for blocks on the sparking axle. I spent the rest of the morning hand-grinding meat for the sausage and nearly ground my thumb off in the process. The *coquelets* I ordered from the butcher still had feathers, which was unheard of, and heads and feet, which was normal. Everything else was stupidly labor intensive but went smoothly. By seven-thirty, when the food was either done or in the oven, I was so exhausted I wanted nothing more than to sleep on the kitchen floor. Unfortunately, I still needed to shower and dress, and there was only an hour before our guest was due. I sat on alert, ready to start snoring, until he arrived at 10:30 P.M., two hours late. He had a lovely bouquet of flowers, but offered no apology for his tardiness.

I served the individual leek and homemade sausage-stuffed *coquelets* with brute cider gravy, the tiniest string beans in the world, and a pumpkin soufflé that I made from scratch, like a slave girl. It cost a fortune in ingredients and took nine solid hours to prepare. Our guest rewarded Thibault, who had done absolutely nothing, with the only compliment: "Very good meal, much better than the hamburgers I thought she'd make."

The day I decided to admit I was not impressed by anything that could be modified with the word *Parisian,* Lucas and I had huddled in a phone booth for over two hours watching haggard Eastern European prostitutes jump into hatchbacks.

Prostitute watching was one of my favorite pastimes for two reasons. One, there were more prostitutes than pigeons in Paris. The male population of the city must have been the horniest or most depraved on Earth. And two, men constantly mistook me for a prostitute, which was odd because I didn't purposely do anything to encourage their advances. I dressed conservatively, never sat around in a parked car, and only loitered in the most acceptable places. Even when I was obviously pregnant, waiting at the bus stop during commuter hours, men approached me and asked that familiar question, *"Combien?"*

In the beginning I was too confused by the language to be offended. "How much for what? A bus ticket?" After a while, however, I understood their intentions perfectly and sought to humiliate them: "Too expensive for a man who rides the bus."

Eventually, I stopped being offended. When they asked I either pretended not to hear, or just told them I wasn't a hooker and went back to reading *The Economist*. I didn't get upset or raise my voice.

One day, as I waited on a bench for my mother-in-law outside the church of St. Sulpice, a man in a suit and Burberry overcoat asked me how much to *sucer sa bitte,* suck his *bitte.* Until this day, schools and churches had been my safe zones. I was caught so off guard he had to repeat his question.

"Suck your what?" What else could it be?

"*Ma bitte.*"

A new word: *bitte,* pronounced like the root vegetable, beet. I explained to the man that my company was not for sale and asked him if *bitte* was indeed feminine, as its article implied. He confirmed the femininity of the male sex organ and laughed when I shook my head lamenting that I'd never figure out this crazy language. He even sat next to me and explained the nuances of *l'argot,* French slang, before wishing me well and heading off with his briefcase in hand. He seemed like a receptive whoremonger to ask one of my million questions about prostitution, and I instantly regretted letting him leave without at least inquiring what about me, exactly, screamed harlot.

That evening Thibault and I had dinner with his family. His mother had scrounged up a four-course meal of au gratin vegetables, pork with caramelized onions, cheese, and some pear cake thing that was all crunchy on top but moist and warm inside. The meal appeared after twenty minutes of her moseying around, occasionally pushing her perfectly sloppy silver bangs out of her eyes, wearing a Cordon Bleu chef's apron over gray flannel slacks and a cashmere twin set, in what appeared to be an empty kitchen. I had personally searched the cupboards, the freezer, and the basement an hour earlier, to no avail, looking for crackers or dry pasta, or anything to keep me from eating my own arm before we sat down together at 9 P.M.

Thibault and his two brothers drank aperitifs in the living room and teased their father. The room was tastefully packed with antiques, the majority of which had been in the family for many, many generations. Apparently, her grandfather was a count or something, and the good kind, a pre-Napoleon title. This was really exciting news for me until they explained that I was nothing, as common as ever. The title had not perpetuated due to sexist laws and, consequently, there was no ceremony scheduled to place a tiara on my head. It occurred to me, looking through jaded eyes at all these old tchotchkes, that the French are just as materialistic as Americans; it is just that their consumerism happened three hundred years ago. Since then, nobody has had to buy useless, beautiful, crap because they inherit it from their parents.

I was busy feeling clever and only listening halfheartedly until I heard, "Well, I may be like you, Papa, but I don't have your big *bitte*!"

I snapped to attention.

"Because you are twenty-four years old! I had no *bitte* at all back then."

White people are insane. This was simply not a conversation you would EVER hear in a black household. Thibault saw my aghast expression and asked what was the matter.

"Did your brother just say he doesn't have your father's big *bitte*?" I asked.

"What!?"

I repeated what I had heard.

"Not *bitte*, *bide*," he explained. "*Bide*, tummy, paunch." Now everyone was laughing at me. Explaining that I'd learned the word from "one of the men who wanted to buy sex from me" quelled the laughter, but not in a good way. I didn't care, though, being so relieved that while the cultural divide was still enormous, the racial divide wasn't quite as wide as I'd thought.

chapter three

Even though I was in my thirties, a mother and wife, the French couldn't separate my ignorance of their language from a general ignorance of how things in the world work. If my language skills were those of a six-year-old, then despite my adult body, I must actually be six years old. All the rude liberties people take with children they started taking with me. A woman on the bus told me to stop biting my nails because it was disgusting and then looked appalled when I said that her body odor mingled with the smell of designer imposter perfume was also disgusting. My brother-in-law tried to tell me about this strange, exotic plant from the orient called bamboo, and how to roll pairs of socks together for tidy storage, as if in the infantile world where I lived socks were nothing more than hand puppets.

All of this not being taken seriously and the inability to communicate were just an annoyance until I became somebody's mother. As a mother I needed respect and credible answers to my child's naive little questions. A responsible French mother knows her son should not hang out at the ice rink because it is a turf peopled by thugs and hooligans. She knows if she sees her son in a public restroom he's not taking a leak; he's taking drugs. She knows that contrary to logic, American-style swim trunks are way more embarrassing than a bikini Speedo. It was my job, for the sake of my son, to get a grasp of this culture.

Thibault tried to explain things to me; but they were rarely the nuances I needed. He never warned me that Parisians consider store-bought desserts more impressive than home-baked ones; so I wasted hours making things like pumpkin soufflés and linzer tortes with berries I gathered myself. He did not explain that the more complicated grammatical construction for asking a question was way less elegant, and significantly more coarse-sounding, than the simple form. So, I ran around verbally exhausting myself and sounding just as wretchedly common as I was.

Plus, Thibault's childhood memories were so random and disjointed that they weren't very useful and I wondered if he truly remembered them or if he'd learned them from a photo album. When I asked him about elementary school all he could tell me was that the kids wore slippers in the classroom and hung their coats in cubbies so they wouldn't catch lice from one another . . . and there was a Japanese boy. He also liked his leather book satchel that smelled like saddle soap. He didn't remember when he learned to read, when test-taking and dictations began, if they had recess, when they learned cursive, if they brought snacks, had animals, or finger-painted. It was all a big blur.

He suffered from the curse of the privileged: the inability to recognize the gift. And having parents who provided and did exactly as they were supposed to do so your individuality could reveal itself at your discretion was a privilege. He was still nestled securely under his parents' wings, and took advantage of his invisibility when out of the nest. Nobody ever challenged him, or ridiculed him, or waited for him to make mistakes. Everything from the baguette sticking out of his armpit to his pouting lower lip, to his unpronounceable, mostly silent-lettered medieval name said "I belong." And he'd never had to deal with the adversity of being a minority, or a foreigner, as I had, and his son soon would. Thibault would teach Lucas man things by example; but all those things you have a mother for, all the details like party favors and framed artwork, and having sleek little *chausson*, not puffy-red *pantoufle* to wear in the classroom were left to all-American me. It was my responsibility to navigate the French social, educational, and class system for my child.

The first thing I needed to do was start socializing my child *à la française*. Since I had no idea how to do that I decided to hire professionals and put Lucas in the local public nursery.

The child care system is so overburdened in Paris that the only way to get service is to constantly harass the administrators. This I learned from an administrator herself. When I added Lucas' name to the waiting list she took both my hands—an uncharacteristically intimate gesture for a Parisian—and looked me in the eye. "If you really, truly want little *Loo-KAH* to learn with our school," she said, "you must call me every day and remind me who you are. Say, 'This is the black American with the garish, orange jacket. My son is still interested.'" I did as I was told, an uncharacteristic gesture for me, and called the school twice a day, every day, until they found a place for him.

With all my free time, I needed to get a job. Finding one

was easy for a native English speaker with a college degree and a work visa. It required just one phone call and I was offered a position as an executive language trainer. With things falling into place so easily, I felt confident I could tackle one last little problem: my comically askew breasts. They hardly allowed me the professional appearance required for my soon-to-be role as a member of civilized society.

Anyone who's ever breast-fed, or spent any time around a breast-feeder, knows how crazy lactating can be. Nipple size and food-making capability aside, lactating breasts behave oddly. One minute they are huge, the next minute deflated, then rock hard, then lumpy. They squirt milk in the shower or soak your shirt when a baby cries on television. One of mine was huge, throbbing, covered with a red rash, and radiating enough heat to defrost a frozen lamb shank in ten minutes. It was like an unpredictable little alien I carried around. Even in the kooky world of milk-making tits, this one worried me.

I stopped breast-feeding as soon as I put Lucas on the school waiting list, but even after two weeks, my engorged breast was so sensitive it hurt to shower. The French doctors had no useful advice for me. Four physicians, including one breast specialist, had come up with nothing better than applying a waxy poultice to "draw out" the soreness, and a ten-day cycle of antibiotics (which I later learned were for respiratory infections).

Paris was cold and boring. I was tired of feeling culturally retarded, stepping in dog feces, and explaining why my baby looked white. I had three weeks before my job started. This was the perfect opportunity to go home to California, remind my child that outside of northern Europe the sun radiates not just light but heat, and maybe see a real doctor about my boob. I bought two plane tickets, kissed my husband good-bye, and took Lucas to visit his loud, black American family.

chapter four

Rebecca, one of my closest friends since high school, picked us up from the San Francisco airport. We'd only been gone a few months, but during that time she managed to lose fifty pounds. I looked at her funny, thinking maybe she'd highlighted her curly blond hair, and then asked if she'd cut it. She frowned and turned her back to me. "Where's your giant ass?" I asked. She beamed. Then she told me all about what she'd done with her ass on the drive to my parents' house.

The neighborhood looked especially ritzy that evening with all the seasonless California landscaping and chandelier-lit windows. The streets were empty except in front of my parents' house. They must have been hosting a dinner party and I knew from the collection of cars that the usual characters were there. I carried the baby and Rebecca rolled my one bag. It was smaller than her ass used to be and I feared I'd under-packed for this trip.

Through the dining room window I could see the caterer running back and forth, playing the role my mother used to play before she retired from homemaking. And my mother was sitting at the table, a sight I still hadn't gotten accustomed to, drinking a glass of wine and rolling her eyes at my father who had a reference book in front of him. (Usually she drank her wine and rolled her eyes while standing.) He was holding his finger in the air asking someone to be patient, clearly about to support his point with published documentation.

The gesture of holding his finger like that was immortalized in an eighteen-inch-tall wooden statue he had in his den. It was just the hand, index finger erect, roughly carved. My whole life I thought that statue was just my father being self-referential. Then, one Thanksgiving, my sister asked him where on Earth he got that crazy thing.

"Well, there was an artist in Korea who made similar statues in the bird position," my father said, flipping his middle finger away from everyone, as though it were a loaded gun. "I asked him to make me one with the index finger. Because as a urologist I do rectal exams."

Growing up, about 90 percent of my family's interactions took place around the dinner table. There were always the five of us, my parents, brother Douglas, sister Angela, and myself, and usually one or two of our friends. Sitting down at the table ensured you would receive a square meal and an education, usually in the field of semantics.

If you brought somebody to dinner it meant you could send him or her to the dictionary instead of going yourself. Guests often didn't know how to hide their ignorance when my father used words like *miscreant* or *malingerer* usually to describe my brother, and ended up getting shipped off to the den where the dictionary sat open on a book stand, the finger statue on the red shag carpet next to it. They were required to look up the word and report back the definition.

We were allowed to voice any opinion we wanted as long as

we could support it. And we got points if we used advanced vocabulary. "Mr. Munroe (the Scottish headmaster at my school who actually insisted we called him Headmaster) is a jerk."

"Why do you say that today, Meredith?"

"Because last week he told Drea she couldn't wear lipstick but she could wear lip gloss and then today he made me wipe off my lip gloss that wasn't even colored, but smelled like root beer, which he said was *'oon-beak-omun,'* on his snotty handkerchief." My father looked unimpressed. I tried to save myself. "His rules are capricious!"

"He is capricious. His rules are inconstant."

We talked about everything except sex, money, and feelings. Unlike some of my friends whose fathers would tease the kids for "whacking off" or being "horny," my parents never used that language or even came close to that subject matter. They never told us how much my father earned, and they never said we couldn't afford something. It might be too expensive, but that was the intrinsic nature of the item, not a reflection of our financial situation. And if we had issues with each other (like when my mother humiliated me at Macy's girls' department shopping for my very first bra, saying to the clerk, "For God's sake, she doesn't actually need a bra, she just needs two little triangles tied to a string!") we coped by repressing our emotions. Despite our African Americanness, we were typical WASPs.

But a big part of being in or around my family was living under the premise that we were all geniuses in the process of improving ourselves. This held true even for my brother, who through a series of destructive misdemeanors sealed in his juvenile file, did his best to convince us he wanted nothing more than to be a quadriplegic jailbird. My father did not send you to his multiple-volume *Webster's* because you were stupid, but because he assumed you had decent intellectual acumen and that increased vocabulary would only better your articulation. Conversation was never dumbed down. You won some points and lost others, but regardless, loaded the dishwasher feeling challenged and respected, not humiliated and demeaned. Nobody ever interrupted your monologue on the Japanese aesthetic to explain what bamboo was.

After months of communication deprivation in France I desperately wanted to join this dinner party conversation. I wanted to get the jokes and allusions, and make puns. So I let myself in, greeted everyone, and tried to say something worth hearing. But my brain, after twenty-four sleepless, exhausting hours traveling with a one-year-old, was incapable of anything better than "It is being near twenty-one hour, is it not?" To which my father responded, "Go to sleep. You're speaking English like a second language."

Rebecca, who'd been a frequent guest at our table and endured years of my father's standards, knew that I couldn't keep up in my present state of mind. She nudged me toward the stairs, briefly helped me get settled in my sister's room, and went home to her own family.

I lay down on the bed next to Lucas and shut my eyes. We were directly above the dining room and I could hear everything through the floor. "The metric system is logical, for one thing . . . Republicans . . . 'No one becomes depraved all at once.' Juvenal . . . Hutus and Tutsis, those cats have issues." Old-school slang and politics lulled me to sleep.

Minutes later my mother shook me awake, encouraging me to change out of my airplane clothes and put a fresh diaper on the baby. As I undressed and she slipped Lucas into his pajamas without waking him, I showed her my chest. "That doesn't look right. Go downstairs and show your father."

"I'm not showing Daddy my boob in the middle of your party."

"They're all doctors."

"Of chemistry, and orthopedics."

"Lawrence is a gynecologist!"

"He's eating."

"Well, then, call your own doctor. That really doesn't look right."

Advice like this coming from Eloise Norton was very worrisome. My mother is an underreactor. As far as she is concerned, there are few nonsocial reasons, ever, to see a doctor. When my brother had spinal meningitis she told him he just needed a nap. When I lost twenty of my one hundred and ten pounds within three weeks of returning from Guatemala, she refused to drive me to the hospital, saying that I should be happy my young metabolism was so fast. I'd miss it (and the six-foot tapeworm) when I got older. It was a strange idiosyncrasy in an otherwise extremely devoted and nurturing woman.

Only once before had she taken me to the doctor for anything other than checkups and protruding broken bones. One morning in high school, I woke up with a rash so severe my eyes had swollen shut. My lips were as inflated as inner tubes, and my tongue stuck out like one of those fetal pigs you dissect in biology class. Mom took one look at me in my school uniform as I caught, in a cupped hand, the saliva pooling around my teeth and spilling over my lower lip, got her keys, and drove me to the pediatrician's office. She never expressed concern at whatever horrible disease might have caused these hives. She just kept repeating how unbelievable it was that I intended to leave the house with my face looking like that. Had I no vanity at all?

The lack of concern of the doctors in France had been infuriating on a professional level, but personally comforting. Of the four doctors I saw in France, only one had ordered further tests, and those, he said, were only valuable in that they might make me feel better. I figured the problem would just work itself out and my breasts would go back to normal eventually. But my mother's advising me to see a doctor immediately for easily camouflaged symptoms was concerning enough that I got up, called the hospital's urgent care hotline, and made an appointment for the next day with my ob/gyn.

Less than twelve hours later I sat on the table waiting for the doctor, feeling like a kid, with my feet dangling about a foot from the floor. In France, at this point in an exam, I'd be frantically reviewing vocabulary words or composing sentences in my head so I'd sound fluent when I stuttered them. But here, in the familiar setting of my own language and culture, I picked at my cuticles and tried to get a raisin skin out from between my teeth.

When the doctor arrived we exchanged pleasantries and I gave her a little background. Before opening the half gown I warned her not to laugh when she saw how lopsided my breasts were. I don't know what about lopsided breasts this professionally trained physician would have found funny. She was hardly some fourteen-year-old boy copping a feel to impress his buddies. But she humored me, promised not to laugh and didn't. I immediately wished she had. Instead, she grimaced, wrinkled her previously adorably freckled nose, picked up the phone, and called the surgery department. That was at 9:15 A.M.

By two o'clock I had seen the surgeon, gotten a skin biopsy, had an ultrasound and mammogram, been scheduled for a stereotactic needle biopsy, and wished a nice weekend.

At one point, while waiting in the lab, a nurse came to escort me to see a second surgeon who'd been called out of the operating room. With so much eager attention I knew there couldn't be anything really wrong. The one time I saw a girl almost die from dehydration, a fairly dramatic death filled with eye-bulging convulsions, the doctors had done nothing at all. They stood around chatting until she became unconscious and stopped moving. That, they explained, was a much better time to insert an IV. If little attention meant lots of urgency, then lots of attention meant little urgency. Them saying that my symptoms were nothing and that it was just easier to get all this done before the weekend further supported this. It sounded like mastitis, they said, a blocked milk duct gone untreated due to the misdiagnosis of those four French doctors. They'd called in the specialist, and were being extra thorough because this hospital had never seen such an advanced case. It seemed plausible and I spent the last totally carefree weekend of my life.

chapter five

My sister Angela's photo albums are thematic. Her recipes are typed. She has made quilts for each holiday. Angela has many eye shadow and lipstick options arranged in a drawer. One of my clearest memories is watching my sister paint her nails in two tones of glossy pink and then looking down at my own nails, bitten raw and painted with Wite-Out. Deep gouges, as though I'd dragged my fingertips across asphalt, which I probably had, were begrimed with two shades of dirt.

My sister made her braces look so glamorous and sophisticated that I wrapped my teeth in tinfoil and craft wire trying to look like her. When she left the house I snuck into her room and tried on her bras. Then I lounged on her bed, leafed through her *Seventeen* magazine, and pretended to gossip with her fast, side-ponytail-wearing friends.

Angela's typical greeting to me was, "Get out of my room, Pigpen, you're getting everything dusty!" She often talked about her future bachelorette apartment and how I would never be allowed in the door. It wasn't because I was four years younger and hopelessly unstylish; it was that I was a rodent breeder and left a trail of guinea pig pellets and hamster droppings wherever I went. Once, after begging her to come into my room, she found a petri dish of moldy skin. Had she not made such a production of shaving her legs I wouldn't have had reason to try shaving my own. And, I wouldn't have had the slug-shaped swath of skin to put in the petri dish in the first place.

By the end of college I'd recovered from my filthiness. Mostly, it was exposure to other truly filthy people that cured me. One guy on my freshman floor never changed his sheets all year. Another girl kept her finger- and toenail clippings in a mason jar. I refused to let myself be grouped with these people.

When the family came to visit my dorm room right before graduation my sister looked around in disbelief and started rifling suspiciously through my drawers of folded turtlenecks and shelves of alphabetized books. She even looked under the bed, something I figured she'd never do again after finding my cockatiel's severed foot years earlier. She was just starting to relax when I slipped a coaster under my brother's sweaty can of Mountain Dew. "It's just that the water leaves rings," I said. Angela jumped back, grabbed the closest weapon she could find—a five-foot-long painted Aborigine rain stick—jabbed it in my face, and screamed, "What did you do with my sister?!" followed by the soothing sound of spring showers.

After that she invited me to her apartment for the first time ever. When I didn't burn anything or cover it in dung Angela lifted the ban on socializing with me. But even ten years later, after hundreds of hours in her personal space, I still considered myself privileged to be allowed in her home. So, when she invited Lucas and me to spend the weekend at her house, I eagerly accepted. Immediately after my whirlwind of doctor appointments I grabbed my boy, jumped in the car, and rushed to Sacramento, which is not exactly the kind of town one goes rushing to. It's a sort of nondescript city surrounded by tract houses and farmland. It's like a little bit of Texas in California. People from the San Francisco Bay Area tended to look down on the state's humble capital until the real estate situation went berserk and they realized it was the only place they could afford to buy a house.

My sister and brother lived within five minutes of each other in what was either suburban Hell or Heaven, depending on your perspective. Their neighborhood was preplanned down to the roof shingle color and speed bump placement. The streets were lined with tiny matching trees and SUVs were parked in every driveway until sundown, when, for purely aesthetic reasons, the Neighborhood Committee encouraged homeowners to keep their cars out of sight and in garages.

The car situation in general was nuts. In Paris, I had walked a hole right through the sole of my shoe. In Sacramento, driving everywhere was mandatory even though every possible retail and entertainment outlet was within walking distance. The only way to be outside and avoid a neighborhood watch call to the police was to put on sweats and jog. Walking five blocks to the supermarket because you wanted to save gas or needed time to think was unpermissibly strange.

My brother, Douglas, was no longer the rich, skinny black kid who fancied himself a petty thug. Surprisingly, he'd become a rather strapping, principled attorney who found the neighborhood consistent with his new image as a respectable professional and family man. Plus, he really enjoyed driving, even with a license. He'd have preferred to live on a golf course, but other than that, and his fear that the Arabs next door were a terrorist cell, he and his wife seemed content.

My sister, Angela, with her SUV and scrapbooking parties, should have been well situated but managed to hate the area and feel out of place. She had all sorts of reasons, but the real problem was that the community created a feeling of false affluence. The houses looked way more expensive than they were. This disparity seeded a fundamental suspicion of her neighbors that when fed by the alarmist media developed into outright distrust. Distrust bred contempt, and once my sister was filled with contempt there was no talking her out of it.

I, however, loved the sparkling newness and convenience of the place. I loved the Starbucks, and the Jamba Juice, and riding a block and a half in a car so tall I felt like a truck driver. For two days I played with my niece and nephews, drank coffee that didn't curl up my tongue, planned my son's birthday party, and actually complained about my hair. We watched hours of HGTV without subtitles and Angela smothered Lucas in auntie-kisses. They might not have laughed, but nobody corrected my jokes or mocked me for wearing track pants out to breakfast. The waitress at IHOP even showed me a picture of her grandson, a redheaded black child just like my own. It was the vacation I'd been looking for, a respite from being foreign.

chapter six

The next Wednesday, I went for the core biopsy. Some microcalcifications were found on my mammogram and although they could indicate precancerous growth, they probably didn't. This was the second time anyone had mentioned cancer. The first time was a French breast specialist who glanced at my breast and said, "Well, it definitely isn't cancer."

I was strangely eager to have my stereotactic biopsy, mostly because the machine fascinated me. It is, in essence, a robot. You lie facedown on a table with your boob protruding through a trap door. The breast gets clamped tight, uncomfortably so, inside an X-ray device, exactly like for a mammogram. Once you're positioned properly, with your neck craned unnaturally and your kneecaps balanced against a sharp edge, a metal probe is inserted into your breast. Guided by the mammogram picture, this probe is a robotic arm. From it, little razor-sharp knives core slivers of flesh for diagnosis. It sounds like a torture device, but the process was surprisingly entertaining.

I was so entertained, in fact, that I didn't even mind the faceless doctor's inability to introduce himself. He just moseyed in, turned off the lights, and started stabbing me with all kinds of little pokers, without a word of hello.

Throughout the procedure I asked question after question.

His answers were always the kind that got you an F in Spanish class, the short-as-possible kind, and the silent kind. "How many of these have you done? What type of software does this thing use? How precisely can you guide the probe? Are you married? What would happen if we had an earthquake or lost power?" He didn't respond to the last question. I asked again, "What would happen if we lost power?" With still no response, I tried to sound technical. "Can you manually extricate me from this machine?" He excused himself and left the room. I was touched by the sudden surge of manners.

"Sweetie," the nurse whispered, "you should never ask questions you don't want to know the answers to." Then she picked something out of my hair, patted my back, and said, "I'll go see what's keeping the bastard."

Left alone, my neck rapidly stiffening, I began to fall into one of my unfriendly brain episodes. These are usually harmless fantasies about finding myself in ridiculous circumstances, such as how long would I live if the only food left on Earth was parsley? I hate parsley. I hate the smell of parsley especially. If I managed to swallow it, how long could it sustain me? But this time, my unfriendly brain was fixated on an earthquake happening with me pegged to this table. I would be forced to tear my breast free like that hiker who cut off his own arm when it got trapped under a boulder.

How much pain would I be willing to endure to save my life? Or my child's life? Would I jump into a tank of sharks to rescue Lucas or would I stand teary eyed on dry land blowing kisses and waving good-bye? I think that for Lucas I would indeed jump into a tank of sharks, but not into a tank of squid.

I would fight lions, but not hyenas. The location of the pain would also be very important. Anything affecting my knees—like bending them backward—would be out of the question. Cutting into my stomach or torso is fine, but the backs of my arms or legs would not be okay. I couldn't do anything involving my eyelids. But my boobs? They hardly belonged to me since Lucas was born. I barely recognized them most days, they were so juglike and in the way. I could definitely pull myself out from the probe. That settled, I fell asleep.

Later that morning, I was ushered into the office of the surgeon, Dr. Ree. First she said, "Hello," and then she said, "You have cancer." She took out a pad of paper, wrote "Inflammatory Breast Cancer" across the top of it, and underlined the words. Under that she printed "Chemotherapy," with an arrow pointing down to "Double Mastectomy." Next to that, in parentheses, she put, "No Reconstruction." And then another arrow pointing down to "Radiation."

Why would this woman who didn't even know me make a joke like this? But Dr. Ree, whose child-sized body bent toward me from her chair, offering an ageless, flawless face, was not laughing and neither was the breast care coordinator. She sat erect, hands folded, with the good posture of the newly pregnant. They were both looking at me with these absurdly long and sympathetic faces that were so effectively sympathetic I wondered if they practiced in front of the mirror. I became more interested in their expressions than in what they were saying. First their faces were sad: *What awful news*. Next they were sympathetic: *We know this is hard for you*. Then determined: *We'll work together and get you through this*. Now, alarmed by my lack of response: *She must be in shock*. And finally, relieved, when the tears started flowing: *Thank God,* their faces said. *She isn't dead on the inside*.

Two strangers had just witnessed the most intimate moment of my life. It was worse than being walked in on while losing your virginity or giving birth in front of a stadium of people. Those acts, by definition, involve other people. Death is really the only thing you do alone, no matter who is there to hold your hand. These spectators watched as I visualized my death, with probable accuracy, for the first time. And the picture was so banal. I was destined for something greater: an assassination, a sacrifice. Plebeian cancer is how it would all be cut short? I'd never play Rummikub with Bill Clinton or have my own self-titled sitcom and theme song? My son wouldn't know his mother? I'd just be that unphotogenic woman pawing at him in all those pictures.

Bad news should be delivered privately. You should sit in a soundproof room with a mirror and a box of tissues. When you're ready, a piece of paper slips through the door. You turn it over and read: *"Sterile"* or *"Nobody likes you"* or *"Herpes Simplex II."* When you are ready, you emerge and fall into the embraces (maybe reluctant, depending on your diagnosis) of strangers.

Dr. Ree continued to talk, something about blood tests and a shortcut to the lab. "What?" I asked her. She explained again. "What?" She drew another diagram. I looked at it, perplexed. "What?" She told me not to worry about it.

The problem was that as Dr. Ree held my hand in her office all I could think was: "She touches people's internal organs with those hands. She uses those hands to wash her hair." I felt the same awe as when I realized that men always have their penises with them, hidden in their pants, even when they aren't using them. Then I went outside to wait for my father, and his penis, to pick me up.

Intense irritation set in almost immediately as I waited in the blazing sun in front of the hospital. The usual characters milled about: a clove-smoking teenager sat reading a hardcover book; an old man shuffled across the street taking random, huge steps. A goddamned mime, in jeans and a T-shirt with a white painted face, headed straight toward me. I watched him approach, look at his watch, grimace, look at the building behind me, at the building across the street, and then at a piece of paper pulled from his pocket. "Where the fuck is Medical One!?" he screamed silently at nobody in particular. I directed him to the building nearby and realized that, lost or not, we are always in character. We are what we are. Then he tripped over an invisible curb and walked away.

I needed five minutes to myself, five minutes with no audience, where I could make all of those hideous, agonized faces one makes during a breakdown. I could have sat happily in my own car in the cool, dark parking lot, bawling my bloody eyes out. Instead, I listened when I was told not to drive myself to hear this news and was now forced to add *sunburned forehead* to my list of ailments and compress all my emotions into tensely crossed arms and an arhythmically tapping foot.

I had just been told that I had only a 40 percent chance of being alive in five years. I needed a double mastectomy. I would never win any wet T-shirt contests. I'd never get nipple erections and I was about to lose all of my hair. Paris wasn't demoralizing; this fucking vacation was demoralizing.

I told my father in the car on the ride back to the house. His shock manifested as a general confusion of traffic priorities. He looked back and forth again and again at every intersection, the way one does when driving in a foreign country. When we got home he told my mother and immediately burst into sobs. I just closed the door, not needing the outward display of hysteria.

Finally alone, I sat in my sister's old bedroom. My mother had converted Angela's room to a closet-slash-guest room and erased all traces of her daughter's former occupancy. My own childhood room was just across the hall. I never stayed there when I visited, even though it would have made more sense. It too served as a guest room, but all my old furniture was gone, replaced by heirlooms from my grandma's house.

I lived in that room for fifteen years, spent thousands of hours there playing or being punished for various obnoxious behaviors. I'd chosen the wallpaper, now painted over, and the carpet, now ripped up. The closet that once held my ice hockey uniform and Gloria Vanderbilt jeans now housed a few board games, some bridesmaid dresses, and a big woolly sweater my grandmother always wore when she came to visit.

Where the fuck was my stuff? I vaguely remembered blowing up my dollhouse with an M80 firecracker. My dresser was destroyed from years of using the drawers as a ladder. My fish tank? My Habitrail? There must have been fifty hamsters buried in the yard. Where was all that crap? At some flea market, displayed pathetically on a folding table, like that photo

album I once bought? Pages and pages of thoughtfully organized family photos, an entire family forgotten, their camping
trips and potty training on display for anyone with seventy-
five cents and two inches of shelf space.

Where had those people gone? It wasn't so old, that book.
It had petting zoos, Mickey Mouse balloons inside of balloons,
bell-bottoms, lots of ivy, carnations, and places I recognized. I
could probably find myself in the background if I looked hard
enough. There at the zoo, back against the fence, with a wild-
eyed goat violently slurping the feed out of my Dixie cup.

One day I would be gone. One day soon, and not long after
that there wouldn't even be anyone to miss me. All the stuff I
dragged around, carefully protected—my social security card,
address book, the bookmark my niece made me—soon enough,
all this would be abandoned junk.

Thibault's call to hear about my appointment interrupted
my pity party. I told him to hold on to his hat because Meredith had cancer. The hesitation before he started to blubber
meant that he hadn't understood the first half of my sentence,
but the second half was perfectly clear. I could tell from the
muffled echo that he was in our long hallway, probably lean-
ing his head against the chenille wallpaper like I'd asked him
not to do a hundred times. It was the first time I had heard
him cry.

"Should I come home?" I asked.

"Are you joking? These stupid damned French shitfucker
doctors goddamned sorcerers! How many of these bitch sons
said to you nothing is wrong? *Putain!* No French doctor will
touch you!"

"Chill out, Furio. That is really sexy and all, but we need to think about this. We live in Paris."

"So what, you want to do this in French? This is serious. *You* need to understand, every word." Translation: my appointments would be in French, a language I spoke very poorly and often didn't understand at all. I would be assisted by my husband, who, although bilingual, inexplicably fails to translate key pieces of information. Sometimes when watching French movies I'll miss a line and ask him what the character said. His typical response is, "This movie is about spies" or "They're speaking French." Such vagueness could cause serious problems in a health care situation.

"And everything takes forever here. You've been in the United States less than a week and already had something like twenty appointments." Meaning: I would have to build my own team of unrelated doctors and outsource for support services such as laboratory testing, X-rays, and chemotherapy. I'd have had to ask for referrals, wait for approvals, and generally waste significant amounts of time on bureaucracy, the French national pastime. In a country that counts 10 percent of its population as functionaries, considerable time and energy would be spent riding buses all over the city picking up and delivering paperwork that could easily be centralized electronically by my U.S. HMO.

"What doctor will you see, the one who gave you the homeopathic cream or the one who said most women have two sizes of breasts?" Granted, even if language and bureaucracy were no problem, I was convinced that every single doctor in the entire country was incompetent. After all the smug misdiagnoses and placebos I'd been given at the hands of French physicians, I had more faith in a troop of trained chimpanzees.

"I tell you right now, there is no fucking way you are coming back to France for treatment," Thibault said. "I will come to you."

Thibault rarely made unilateral decisions or outbursts of any sort. I didn't have the heart, or the will, to oppose him.

The life I'd just settled into, the kitchen where my pots hung, the bathroom with my mouthwash and sloppily folded towels, my washing machine that only held two T-shirts and took ninety minutes minimum to run a load, my PAL exercise tapes, and my new placebo mommy group friends I was pretending to like were all behind me. I'd never see them again. Had I known, I would have stopped and placed a bookmark, taken a mental snapshot of the place rather than rushing out of it with the baby on one hip, paltry luggage over my shoulder. I would have picked up the mail from under the welcome mat rather than kicking it back through the door before I slammed it behind me. I would have said good-bye to my enviable life.

chapter seven

Thibault arrived in San Francisco the next day looking knackered and tear dehydrated. His pale skin was sallow, and his blue eyes were rimmed with red. Even his usually unruly hair looked defeated. After we'd spoken on the phone he called his parents, threw some things in a duffle bag, and went to the airport. He took the first flight to San Francisco and met me wearing the same clothes he'd worn to work the day before.

At baggage claim he folded himself around me, squeezing tightly, and buried his face in my neck. I thought, "God, people must really think we're in love." Then he held my hand and didn't say anything for the whole ride home.

The next day we met my three doctors with three very different personalities. My outdoorsy ob-gyn with the adorably sunburned nose, Dr. Lowery, had diagnosed me and passed me over to the surgeon, Dr. Ree. Dr. Ree insisted that I call her by her first name, which I never did, and was full of hugs and assuring hand squeezes. She gave me her home phone number and returned my pages immediately, even from the operating room. She seemed to be more concerned for me than I was. Dr. Yuen maintained a professional distance and spoke in measured and precise language. I loved talking to her because she had obviously learned English from a textbook, but was polishing it with the aid of somebody who'd grown up in the

San Fernando Valley. She described my lymph nodes as "totally funky" and said my tumor should be "like, less humongous" after chemo.

My father researched their backgrounds and verified that they all had excellent training and reputations. Despite their youth (none of them was even forty) they were well-regarded leaders in their fields. We hung on every word, wrote down every suggestion, and felt confident. None of them inspired the dread I felt when the specialist was called in to see me about my migraines at the French hospital. When he appeared two security guards pushed him to the door. "There is no free dinner for you in here. Out!" He had to correct them, saying he was a neurologist, not a homeless man.

Time not spent at the medical center was spent wallowing (imagining all the things that weren't going to happen, like me walking in on my preteen son masturbating) and lying to our friends, saying Thibault had flown in for Lucas' birthday party. It would have been much easier to go ahead and tell everyone, not just family, what was happening, but neither of us wanted to ruin Lucas' first birthday. Even though canceling the party would have given us more time to pity ourselves, all the statistics predicted that we might not get another opportunity to celebrate as a family. So instead, we dragged ourselves around town, pretending nothing was wrong besides jet lag, ducking out of conversations into restaurant bathrooms to cry into our hands.

The invitations were shaped like rocket ships, but should have been shaped like martini glasses with a caption of "Bottoms

Up!" The party turned out to be more of a happy hour than anything else. My family, in the WASP spirit we embrace, drank all the alcohol in the house and then went out and bought more. My sister, with Phyllis Diller's delivery, said, "This is the first first birthday I've been to where we should have taken people's keys."

Lucas cried the whole time and clung to me like a tick. My brother and his wife raised suspicions by moping considerably less than usual. When we sang "Happy Birthday" it sounded like a funeral march, so much so that we had to start over, which coaxed the first genuine laugh out of any of us all day. Our guests were confused and their early departures made it clear they regretted coming.

Rebecca had no idea what was going on, so the second everyone else left she cornered me and asked, "What the f-u-k-c (she's dyslexic and her daughter was playing nearby) is going on?"

"I have cancer."

"That explains your lame-ass party."

One of Rebecca's lifelong complaints about me is my persistent lack of emotionalism. The last few days I'd been an emotional wreck, despite my efforts to conceal it. "You got choked up at the gas station." That was when I realized my own extinction would precede fossil fuel technology's. "And that kid, with the crazy 'PIPM' gold teeth. Even I saw they were misspelled and you didn't say anything. You're distracted. I knew something was wrong. And it wasn't no f-u-k-n jet lag." She wiped her eyes. Then she hugged me really tight for extra long.

chapter eight

I was hardly the anxious wreck anyone expected for my first round of chemo, administered one week and two days after I landed at SFO. I had never been afraid of needles, never squeamish. I ate during televised bouts of liposuction or face-lifts. I loved how they violently poked the suction tube under the skin and cut the fat out of an eyelid. Nothing was more satisfying than the dull sound of hammer chiseling live nose bone. At course one, I was the ideal patient. I had huge veins, never flinched, and was full of jokes.

Thibault didn't know what to expect. He'd been rather shell-shocked since arriving and it was obvious by his carefully chosen greeting of "Good morning, I am happy to see you" that he'd promised himself not to say anything today to upset me, including asking questions.

Upsetting me by asking questions was something Thibault had avoided since our very rocky baby homecoming a year earlier. Like many men, my husband was a total ignoramus regarding the baby. When it cried he asked me why. When it shat its diaper he asked me for permission to change it. He began asking me if *he* could go to the bathroom, and if it was all right to have a beer, what time it was when there was a clock right there, and for directions to places he knew perfectly how to find. I suddenly had two babies, something I had never, ever wanted. I applied various negative stimuli to discourage this new behavior. When he pointed to the clearly labeled glass jar of pickles sitting eighteen inches in front of him, a jar that he had chosen and bought himself, and asked me what it was, I simply pinched the back of his arm as hard as I could. He shrieked and didn't ask me another stupid question for almost two days. When I pinched him again, this time for asking me if he could press the button on the elevator, it was hard enough that he didn't ask me questions of any sort for almost a week. The habit was broken and I rarely resorted to the pinching technique again. He either became more resourceful or more comfortable living in his cloud of ignorance.

Since he was afraid to ask for specifics, the only thing Thibault knew about chemotherapy was what he'd seen in movies: intense nausea, vomiting, and pensive walks along the seashore. When the session started, he sat next to me quietly, reserving his energy for the long night that lay ahead. He prepared to stoically hold my shoulders while I hugged the toilet bowl. He would chivalrously lay cold compresses over my eyes.

It turned out he worried for nothing. The chemo wasn't administered like grain to a goose; it wasn't crammed down my throat with a big funnel or forced in any other orifice. After sitting and chatting pleasantly for three hours with an IV stuck in the back of my hand, it was done. I felt so good we went to the Claremont Resort to visit friends and drink virgin mojitos by the pool. Aside from the fact that I'd just injected my body with powerful toxins, it was a lovely day.

Looking out over the view of San Francisco Bay, it occurred to me that only two things had really changed: one, I was still going to die, but my means of death was more probable now that I had cancer; and two, nobody was going to let me pick up the tab for these overpriced drinks. I probably wouldn't have to buy my own drink for months. It didn't mean that one of my old boyfriends couldn't still kill me. I could still get hit by another golf cart, only this time it might mean a broken neck, rather than some cracked ribs and bent clubs. And there was always the giant squid.

Later that evening I started to feel drunk. Not giggly inebriated, but shitface intoxicated, the kind of drunk you get when you drink rubbing alcohol instead of grain alcohol, or at your kid's first birthday party. I took a tiny antinausea pill and within minutes, miraculously, simply felt hungover. I lay down, turned out the lights, and slept dreamlessly until morning. Then I got up and peed the most noxious-smelling urine imaginable. It wasn't even yellow, but grayish-brown, like water emptied from a steam cleaner.

My father, the resident urologist, insisted that I drink as much water as possible. The chemo drug, Cytoxin, is, ironically, a known carcinogen; if not sufficiently diluted it can cause bladder cancer. (The liquid I'd consumed the day before, in various forms of expensive nonalcoholic cocktails, was apparently insufficient.) Even though I drank until my belly felt stretched past capacity, the smell of my urine was so potent it made my eyes water. It slowly evolved into a meaty, rotten odor, slightly sweet and bloody smelling. That lasted for about a week, or a day or two before my next treatment.

I dreaded going to the bathroom. It was like being pregnant again. Only, when I was pregnant I dreaded two things: one, thinking I was finished peeing and then standing up to discover I'd been mistaken; and two, the appearance of the mysterious mucous plug. I had no idea what it actually looked like, but my imagination told me that enough congealed mucus to keep a baby from falling out was probably something I'd enjoy on television but wouldn't want to see hanging from my own vagina.

Cancer treatment brought with it a whole host of images I didn't want to personalize: total baldness, for example. A hairless body has its appeal, but losing eyelashes and eyebrows just looks creepy. My hair could be damaged but it still had to be on my head. I had never even been able to muster the courage to cut it short; the closest I got was baby doll bangs in the sixth grade. One day after my mother dropped me off at school I went into the upper school girls' bathroom and, without the benefit of a comb or brush and using a pair of construction scissors from the first grade classroom, chopped off the front third of my hair. I knew instantly I'd made a huge mistake. My new bangs started to frizz up, and by the time my class was called to the auditorium for pictures I had a triangular patch forming a halo across the crown of my head. It is an image I recall often, whenever I suspect myself of having unrealistic expectations or am considering doing something without the proper tools.

But somehow, despite everything I knew about chemotherapy drugs, I was convinced that my hair wouldn't actually fall out. For fifteen years I'd been relaxing, coloring, texturizing, teasing, blow-drying, hot-combing, and flat-ironing and managed to keep it from falling out. Surely, my overprocessed hair, which always looked awful as a result of the aforementioned abuses, was accustomed to greater hardship than regular hair and would resist the chemo like Wonder Woman's bullet-deflecting bracelets.

It did put up a good fight. When I went in for my second treatment, two full weeks later, the nurses were amazed that the shedding hadn't started. I cleaned and inspected my brush thoroughly every day and never counted more than a handful of hairs. At this rate, I'd have a full head of hair until I was eighty, if I managed to fall into the 40 percent of people still alive after five years.

Tuesday things changed. As I stood in the shower lathering up I noticed an awful lot of hair on my bar of soap, and on my shoulders, and between my toes. I got a comb and started dragging it across my scalp. It was clogged full with each stroke. My scalp tingled. It was strangely satisfying. My hair felt so thin, my skull so close, but when I looked in the mirror I could hardly see the difference. If not for the Pomeranian-sized heap of hair covering the shower drain I would never have believed the shedding had begun.

My mother always hated washing my hair when I was little because it literally took an hour of wrestling to detangle. I was forced to wear tight braids whenever I swam and then rinse the chlorine without undoing them. Once, when left alone with the babysitter, I decided to take out my braids and plunge my head in the filled kitchen sink. The tumbleweed that emerged was so overwhelming that I lost my comb in it. I hid in the coat closet, and ended up falling asleep wedged securely between the safe and a stack of broken umbrellas. By the time my mother woke me with the jabbing heel of her Ferragamo's, my hair had dried and shrunk up into one enormous dreadlock shaped like the continental United States. The detangling was merciless and each stroke of the comb brought another tear streaming down my face. I dared not mutter a sound for fear that my mother, still impeccably dressed in a beige ultra-suede suit with matching knee boots, would give me another reason to cry.

I brought Thibault in to look. He agreed that my hair appeared normal so when I directed his attention to the shower floor his jaw fell open. "Why," he asked, "is everything in this country so big? *Merde.*"

For the next two days I lost outrageous amounts of hair in the shower. I carefully gelled down what remained to hide the mangy bald spots. It was starting to look a little thin, but was more or less unnoticeable until Target. There, in front of the Hello Kitty party invitations, I reached to scratch over my ear and all the hair, clear to my temple, peeled off, like a piece of Velcro. It even made that ripping Velcro sound. Rebecca stared in amazement, and then I peeled off the other one. We stood in the stationery and office supply section holding the two stiff patches and laughed until our cheeks ached.

Later on I took another shower. I combed and tugged until no more hair came free. The back of my head was as slickly bald as a Romanian orphan baby's. The sides were patchy and the top very thin. With so little density, my normally dark brown hair looked really red. Maybe I'd have to stop blaming my husband's grandfather for my son's carrot top.

I spent the rest of the evening trying to look seductive and

batting my eyelashes at poor Thibault. I twisted my sixteen little hairs around my finger, winked provocatively and mouthed,
"Licky, licky." He tried not to cry. I had honestly never, ever,
seen myself look so bad—not when I got stung on the face by
a Portuguese man-of-war, or slept with my forehead sticking
out of my sleeping bag at Girl Scout camp and it got attacked
by mosquitoes. This baldness made me officially the least de-
sirable woman alive.

I woke up the next morning, shuffled into the bathroom to
pee meat and gag, and was shocked and horrified by what I
saw in the mirror. During my sleep I had somehow forgotten
about my hair loss. I could hardly comprehend the pajamaed
orangutan staring back at me.

I walked out to show Thibault and found Rebecca standing
at my open front door. "Your hair is fucked up," she greeted
me matter-of-factly, and then passed me a glass of freshly
squeezed tangerine juice. She shaved off what was left of my
ego and Thibault's id while I held Lucas on my lap. I thought
he'd be traumatized but he didn't care at all. He kept lunging
for the little disposable razor to shave my head himself.

Thank God for Lucas, my little egomaniac. He was so utterly incapable of comprehending this disease that it was almost as if it didn't exist. Cancer was no excuse for not playing
with him, or for being cranky and selfish. The world was still
an ever-expanding and curious place for him. The fact that his
first trip to the beach might be my last was irrelevant. I couldn't
sit there lamenting my circumstances while he was busy growing up.

Lucas' adaptability aside, I was traumatized by my new

baldness. I wasn't just bald; my scalp was gray and mottled and I suddenly looked sick. I felt embarrassed. This wasn't funny at all. I kept touching my head, still sensitive and stinging from the razor, and wishing I could disappear. Not be dead, but invisible. I was on the verge of tears for days.

When Rebecca found me in a corner at the Puma Outlet trying on a black wool cap and came at me with open arms it was the first time since skinny-dipping in snow runoff that I welcomed a hug. Since the diagnosis, all the hugs may have been intended to help me, but were really serving the hugger. Suddenly, these embraces were a refuge that I could hide my knobby, gray head behind. I was so ashamed to be contaminated by this ugly disease and have it broadcast so publicly.

My self-consciousness was so debilitating that when I went to buy wigs I actually hid in a storage closet to try on each new style. Baring my head in front of the store clerk was too humiliating. In retrospect, I realize she'd seen all kinds of craziness: people who burned half their hair off freebasing, break-dancers who'd slipped off their linoleum, tall people who habitually scraped their heads on textured ceilings. My little temporary chemotherapy baldness was probably the most normal thing she'd seen all day. Still, I hid behind my sister and avoided eye contact with strangers.

I couldn't even wear the wigs I bought. I looked absurd. As a kid I had loved to wear them. I'd march all over town with a neat little Dorothy Hamill. It would be all lumpy and deformed by my huge braids tucked underneath. I didn't care if people knew it was a wig or not. It was a fun costume. If a strong wind blew and sent my wig skedaddling, my own healthy, lustrous (this was before the heat and chemicals) tangled and twig-filled hair would be revealed.

But my wig fascination deteriorated as the years passed. When I was about twelve, I made the mistake of wearing a fake ponytail to a Jack-and-Jill picnic. Every child of a black professional within a fifty-mile radius converged to scrutinize each other and I was shamelessly outed for sporting fake hair in the pre-blatant-weave-wearing early eighties. After pretending that I didn't care for what seemed like two hundred hours, I hid under the Wild West stagecoach in the kids' playground. It was as good as leaving completely, as no Jack or Jill over the age of six would be caught anywhere as uncool.

And later, in college, my boyfriend Nate managed to yank off my wig at the University Food Market and then denied it ever happening. His performance appeared so artless that only two things kept me from believing him. One, my wig had been firmly bobby pinned to my hair so when he plucked it off at the checkout counter he took a good chunk of my scalp with it. I still had the little patch of uncured leather with the tangle thatch attached in my jacket pocket. Two, at that exact point, I was already fed up with him.

He was living in London and traveling back and forth to New York about every ten days to visit. Because he was "in from Europe" I was obligated to drop whatever I was doing and entertain him. That could mean going to a party with his *Lampoon* friends, where I'd be too afraid to raise my arms for fear my armpits would be smeared with cheese, or watching

Home Alone for the fifth time with his aristocratic Polish grandmother who insisted on speaking any language I could not understand.

After an hour of arguing we went to eat lunch at the Oyster Bar at Grand Central Station. While he and his friends ate oysters and talked about climbing Machu Picchu, I sat and sulked over the events of the morning and devised a way to get out of this relationship. I excused myself to the bathroom and wrote a quick Dear Nate letter. When I returned to the table I slipped it into his luggage and really enjoyed my meal. I don't even like oysters, but I slurped them down gleefully.

I expected him to get back to London, start unpacking, and discover the note. However, British customs intervened. He was stopped at the airport, interrogated for suspicion of working without papers, and given a thorough physical search. Then an immigration officer riffled through his bags and discovered the note. He asked Nate what it was. Nate said he had no idea, and the officer proceeded to read the letter to him. I got a call from England, not twelve hours after the dewigging. He'd been violated, humiliated in front of several customs officers, and dumped by his adorable coed girlfriend. Plus, he'd been forced to sit in a center seat in coach class, wedged between an ancient Arab guy who kept spitting phlegm into his handkerchief and a Chinese man whose waxy suit was saturated with cigarette smoke. Justice had been swift, but I still felt disinclined to wear wigs.

But most of all, needing a wig because my body was so toxic that nothing could live in it just felt pathetic, like a ploy for sympathy or an admission of vulnerability. It never felt practical or, surprisingly, even logical. Seeing myself in a hat of some Laotian woman's shiny black hair was beyond comical. I wasn't fooling anyone. I would be better off trying to convince people I'd grown a coonskin cap. I felt like a walking garage conversion and kept hearing my sister's voice saying, "You can always tell they're converted garages." When I shared this with her, well after the fact, she amended it by saying, "Unless you can't," a nuance that might have made a real difference.

Anyway, I'd developed hot flashes that caused me to tear off any insulating head cover no matter where or when. Take my word for something: people are significantly less horrified when you tear off a hat and reveal a bald head than when you tear off a wig, no matter how phony it looks. One or two incidents of children screaming, or old people walking into lamp-posts, is all it takes to convince a girl of that.

chapter nine

When the hot flashes first began I kept looking up to find the heat lamp focused on my head. I'd be sitting there, doing nothing, exerting no energy whatsoever, and beads of sweat would rise on my forehead and upper lip. Within a few minutes I had armpit rings. "It's hot as hell in here! God almighty! That damn George Bush and his global frigging warming. How do you do this to your own goddamned planet?!" Then it would pass and I'd be temperature appropriate for a few hours.

It didn't take long to realize that unlike most things, this wasn't George Bush's fault. I was the only one sleeping in my underwear yet literally sweating right through my pillow. Ten minutes of online research taught me that there were eight potential causes for my symptoms. Three seemed probable for obvious reasons: cancer, medication, and infection. One seemed likely, just because it sounded karmic: idiopathic hyperhidrosis, an inexplicable overproduction of sweat. (I once rejected this really sweet, really sincere guy after he left a sweaty ass print on my sofa. Had I known he was suffering from hyperhidrosis I might have rejected him more kindly.) And the last four seemed unlikely because they just weren't very interesting: hypoglycemia, hormone disorder, neurological conditions, and menopause.

Perhaps the chemotherapy medication wiped out my

immune system and it was a spiking fever from some raging infection? Or maybe the cancer had spread to my pituitary gland, making me unable to regulate my body temperature? Maybe there *was* a heat lamp on my head. Stranger things had happened.

The same Nate who was stopped at British customs was earlier tormented for an entire school year by his college roommates. Each night they secretly smeared a tiny trace of Limburger cheese in the armpits of his pajamas. The smell was subtle and organic, and it lingered even after he changed his clothes. For months Nate suffered silently, showered compulsively, avoided close contact, and never mentioned his problem to anyone until he sat his roommates down and gravely explained that he was checking into the hospital for a battery of tests to determine the cause, perhaps a glandular disorder, of the peculiar odor they may or may not have noticed. They let him do it, too. It wasn't until they were moving out at the end of the semester that one of the roommates showed Nate what was left of the cheese kept in a Tupperware container on the outside window ledge. He handed it to him and said, "Smell familiar?" Nate hadn't gotten laid all year.

I wasn't wasting a year suffering like this. Perhaps one of my Hell-bound friends was playing a joke, but if not, if these meltdowns had a physiological source, a physician was going to find it. I scheduled an appointment to see Dr. Yuen and explained the problem.

"Totally. That is totally normal. Your ovaries are, like, suppressed by the chemo, as is expected."

"For how long?" I asked.

"Well, permanently."

"My ovaries don't work PERMANENTLY?"

Why the fuck hadn't anyone told me about this? I bit my lip and flared one nostril and for the first time Dr. Yuen saw that I was seriously upset. Not the upset where you sniffle and cry, but the ghetto-style upset where you burn down someone's check-cashing business.

"But Meredith, there was no choice. Without chemotherapy you would surely have died."

Yes, I suppose my dead ovaries were equally useless as suppressed ones, but what about harvesting and freezing my eggs before you pickled them in drugs? What about telling me or asking me and giving me a goddamned choice? Nobody, under any circumstances, had the right to take away my ability to reproduce without at least giving me a heads-up.

She looked really surprised and I briefly thought I might be overreacting . . . fuck that. Maybe patients in their late forties or fifties don't worry about those things, but thirty-four is the new twenty-four as far as having babies nowadays. You simply don't just take someone out of the game as if it is a nonfactor.

I spent a good twenty-four hours staring at Lucas, thanking God I'd had him in the nick of time, and hoping he'd be okay as an only child. Then I considered all his freakish characteristics, like his red hair or unmatching ears, and wondered if they were deliberate or just flukes of nature. Were these traits specific to him, or would all of my spawn be so emblematic? I'd never know.

Suddenly I wanted eighteen children and these doctors had stolen them from me. How to cope? Thibault suggested that I remember the vow I made after gaining nearly eighty pounds and living for five months with a dislocated rib during my pregnancy, namely that I would never, ever, under any circumstances, even if humanity were going extinct, give birth to another child. That did make it easier. Then he asked me to focus on the positives. Menopause meant no periods, no birth control, no monthly mood swings. "No more crazy wife who growls! It is the greatest gift for our family." He could have stopped at no periods. This was indeed a great gift. I started laughing at the women in the feminine hygiene aisle at the drugstore. Poor menstruating slaves to the uterus. Waste your good money on plugging that leak; I'm buying scented bath oils!

chapter ten

Since Lucas' birthday was over there was no longer any reason to keep my situation secret. I, however, was probably the worst person to have been responsible for spreading the news of my illness. Some friends did take it upon themselves to make a few calls, but mostly it fell on me. In the beginning I took people aside and carefully explained the details. "Don't get upset," I said, "but I have some bad news. It's not bad for you, bad for me. I have stage III inflammatory breast cancer . . . there is a forty percent survival rate . . . no, that's not very high . . . yes, I'll need a mastectomy . . . blah blah blah." But soon my statistics were off and my treatment was confused; I couldn't remember what the drugs were called. I started spreading false rumors about myself.

Even worse than the misinformation, my delivery was implausible. After the tenth time of telling the same story it was hard to avoid abridging, or even to sound sincere. Most of my close friends already wondered why I was spending my entire vacation going back and forth to the doctor. They suspected something and, although shocked by the seriousness of the diagnosis, were not caught totally off guard. Their eyes would first squint suspiciously; then, after I assured them it wasn't a lie, they would tear up and hug me longer than I felt comfortable.

Things rapidly became absurd. I told one friend while her

husband was out of the room. She was sitting on the floor, looking like a fallen soufflé, when he came in and asked what was going on. She couldn't speak so I told him, openly laughing at the excessive drama of the situation. The poor guy didn't know what to do. Should he laugh, too?

Then there were the people I ran into around town. They were initially angry that I was home and hadn't called them. One woman said I better have a damned good reason. When I said I was about to start chemo she laughed and then burst into tears in the middle of the street, where I left her. I had to get to the bank before it closed. Although tempted to feel bad about abandoning her there, I couldn't be bothered. There was enough on my mind without adding other people's mourning processes to my plate.

The three worst groups of people to tell were the ones that had heard and didn't know what to say when they saw me, the cancer survivors who expected me to feel some sort of camaraderie, and the pitiers who refused to believe that I wasn't secretly a hysterical, hopeless, vomiting shell of my former self. The latter would approach me with long faces, utterly distraught. They'd shake their heads and hug me too long and say, "How. Are. You. Doing?" When I'd say, in all honesty, that I was fine, they'd look to the sky, nod their heads, and ask for the truth.

Well, the truth was that I was doing great, until I saw their funereal fucking faces. Now, I felt like slapping someone. "No, really," they'd say, "let me know if there is anything I can do for you."

"How's about you stop looking at me like I'm already dead?"

But the people that made me most uncomfortable were the other cancer patients and survivors. They would clasp my hands tightly and demand that I curse this disease, this awful scourge. I tried, but couldn't do it with any heart. Cancer isn't a typical parasite. I didn't catch it sitting on some dirty toilet seat. It didn't burrow between my toes and weave its way to my intestines, diverting all my food and growing to six feet, like the tapeworm I had in Guatemala. That, I could curse, weakly, as my limbs grew more emaciated and my stomach more distended. I was not thrilled with cancer, but I couldn't see myself personifying it and then putting a hex on it like some scorned gypsy lady.

But it seemed so disrespectful to tell another cancer patient, "Let go of my hands, you kook!" that I almost always acquiesced and lazily stamped my feet and said sternly, "Bad cancer!" I felt like an idiot every time, and every time vowed to never do it again. Then some other random bald person would approach me at the grocery store or car wash and rope me into this lame ritual all over again.

Does this happen with any other ailment? Do fellow hemorrhoid sufferers clasp hands and chant, "Die hemorrhoids!"? Do they approach other people walking gingerly or sitting on inflatable o-rings and offer this exercise as a form of empowerment? Were I to chant anything, it would be, "Please, God, don't let this disease make me campy!"

I usually blamed people's bad reactions on youth, meaning they weren't accustomed to their friends' being seriously ill or dying, and shock; I rarely prepared them for the arrival of bad news by assuming a grieved expression. Mostly I just blurted out something like: "Yeah, we were visiting my parents but then I found out I have cancer, so now I'm spending my savings on shoes, lotions, and cheese. How have you been?"

"I quit my job," one person responded. Another asked, after rapidly evaluating the closeness of our relationship, "Ooh, what kind of cheese?" The rest tried mostly not to cry.

In general, people responded exactly as I expected. Only twice was I really shocked. The first time was by a girl I hadn't seen since high school. We had been on the rowing team together, often one seat behind or in front of the other. We were friendly, but it wasn't like I'd ever slept over at her house. When I told her I had breast cancer she erupted with emotion.

"My God, how fucking awful!" she wailed. I put down my scone and looked around at the other people in the café. They were staring in serious concern at this woman bawling next to my table.

For the next fifteen minutes she went on and on about how unfair life is and how brave I was and how she would have given her left nut to help me. Afterward, Thibault asked me, "What is this 'lefnut' she wants to *geeve* you?" When I explained that she was referring to the testicles she didn't have, he wrote her off as a maniac and went back to playing Grand Theft Auto. During her teary purge I deduced that she was under heavy hormonal influence. My conclusion was confirmed by the Midol fact sheet she handed me with her phone number scribbled across it.

My second shock came from one of my parents' close friends, a woman I had known nearly all my life. Carmen was always quirky and drove her own daughters crazy. She'd do things like call in and quit their jobs, or download their credit ratings and tell everybody the scores. But with me she had never transgressed, and I regarded her fondly. When I told her I had cancer she asked me about the side effects. I replied that while they weren't a problem at first, the chemo had lately been interfering with my energy level.

"Well, you've always been a complainer," she said.

chapter eleven

Throngs of people came out of the woodwork to contact me. So many seemed suspicious of my illness that I started to wonder about myself and my own credulity. I'd always been an exaggerator, but never the type to flat out lie about something serious. The ones who visited seemed truly relieved that my head really was bald and my hands covered with tracks. People needed to verify that I wasn't exaggerating and that cancer wasn't just a Meredith word for eczema.

But truly, what was most disturbing about the calls was just how much of my personal medical information people I hadn't spoken to in years managed to dig up. They had details, not just the oh-I-heard-you-were-sick kind of news. They would say things like, "I heard you had breast cancer with a concentration of disease around the right nipple." Cancer had become the new birth story, a subject where people felt perfectly comfortable discussing genitals and asking invasive questions. More than once, I interrupted a phone interrogation on the subject of chemotherapy's side effects, such as vaginal dryness to ask, "Who the fuck is this?" Half the time, it was some acquaintance I'd met once ages ago, but sometimes it was a long-lost connection, and I was freaked out but thankful.

Of all the people who did call, it was the ones who didn't that I kept thinking about. Most of the time the "nonresponse" didn't bother me, but a couple of times I'll admit to

being insulted, and, a third time, really hurt. The guy I was en-
gaged to for three years, who sent greeting cards to my grandmother's bridge friends for Groundhog Day, didn't write me
for months after I knew he knew. When he did write, it wasn't
one of his typically carefully scripted, handwritten novellas
squeezed onto a card made by feet-painters that he'd found at
a crafts fair, but a generic postcard with three unremarkable
lines.

The second guy was another person I dated for a long time
and had known since we were preteens. He was made aware
a month after my diagnosis by a mutual friend, his wife's
obstetrician, while his wife gave birth to their second child.
Granted, it was probably fairly upsetting news to hear while
you're trying to celebrate the birth of your daughter, and probably a reaction your wife won't exactly appreciate as she squeezes
eight pounds of her love for you through her loins, but nonetheless, his call a year later wasn't exactly appreciated either. It was
mostly lameness about how upset he'd been and how it had
taken him a year to work up the courage to call me. It was the
same chicken-shit balllessness that caused our breakup.

And the last person was Maceo, my high school crush first
love, who never called and never wrote and I knew he knew
because I'd sent him many telepathic messages. I could have
honored our adolescence together by having a friend call to
tell him, pretending as though I knew nothing about it. Maybe
she could even call three-way and I'd listen silently as he burst
into tears, ruing our breakup and the wasted years since. Or,
more likely, he'd show no emotion at all, not caring anymore
about some dumb girl he dated as a teenager, and I'd fall into

a pit of despair difficult to explain to my doting husband. His not calling almost made me hate him or, even worse, not love him maniacally anymore.

Far more people resurfaced than remained lost. The most shocking reappearance was my close childhood friend Andrea. We were as close as sisters and endured years of private school together. From the formative ages of nine through fourteen, we were the only black girls in our class. That simple fact brought us together, but our symbiotic personalities kept us together. My eagerness to corrupt, coupled with Andrea's willingness to be corrupted, made us steadfast friends. Luckily, my idea of corruption was making adverbs out of swear words and inserting them in Mad Libs. In our sheltered world recess was spent hiding behind the hedges at the far end of the field doing dickily masked grammar exercises. Andrea always appreciated my crassness and rewarded me with her distinctively booming laugh.

Even though we went to different high schools and she fell in with the "jazz hands" drama crowd, we stayed close and saw each other regularly. I still considered her my best friend a year after we graduated from high school and she called me an Uncle Tom to my face and wrote me off because I refused to join her militant war against "The Man." She'd gone off to college excited and laughing and returned for Christmas vacation with a bitter scowl and the belief that the whole world had conspired to keep black people down. Anyone who didn't fully agree was part of the problem.

I was part of the problem. I did admit that America and much of the Western world was designed for the betterment of white men, but I just thought that if anyone should think the whole world hates them, it should be Jews. Black people have had a rough four hundred or so years; Jews, as a group, have been harassed since they picked a team name a few thousand years ago. Plus, the only people trying to exterminate black people are other black people. White people wanted us around so badly they tried to breed us like livestock. White men, as an institution, have been willing to trample on and exploit their own women and any other race that interferes with their progress. It is a conclusion I came to years ago and have probably spent all of forty minutes thinking about since.

In my whole life I could only pinpoint one undisputable personal case of racism that I knowingly suffered. I was in middle school, probably thirteen years old, and had gone on a ski trip with my friend Amy Hartnett and her church group, Oldham Hall. Oldham Hall was one of those nutty, crunchy, university-based churches designed to keep college students in the pews and away from one-night stands. They had slogans like "Come share a keg of prayers" and "Prepare for your JD (Judgment Day)" and sermons titled "Loving Jesus 101" and "The Physics of the Ascension."

Amy was in the junior youth group, a sort of Sunday school–day camp with college students as counselors. They sponsored outings to football games and things like this ski trip. The place wasn't exactly overflowing with black people. In fact, the few times I went to mass with Amy, after Saturday night sleepovers, I was often the only black person in attendance at all. The same held true for the trip to Squaw Valley.

Our parents had given us each a hundred dollars for the

weekend. We pooled the money and Amy held on to it. That first night, when we arrived at the ski lodge, Amy discovered the money was gone. She freaked out, frantically searched through all her clothing, and then, when she couldn't find it anywhere, accused me of stealing it, saying that I was the only person she knew who'd do such a thing. The fact that I had never stolen anything except for a panda bear hairclip from a drugstore when I was seven was irrelevant. And why would I steal my own one hundred dollars and have to sit in a ski lodge with a Catholic priest all weekend? Amy went crying to one of the counselors who preached to her that sometimes black people didn't have all the things white people had and Amy should look to God to understand this.

Now, my father was a surgeon. I lived in an impressive house in an exclusive neighborhood and I went to the same private school as Amy, although she, unlike me, needed financial aid to pay tuition. Her father was a mediocre real estate agent and her parents rented out rooms in their house. When I asked my father for lift ticket money he just opened his wallet and handed me a hundred-dollar bill. Amy, on the other hand, had begged her parents for the money and then ended up babysitting to raise the last forty bucks.

To add insult to injury, these pious Oldman Hall bastards called an emergency meeting, from which I was excluded, to discuss this situation and pray for me. As they exited the hall, they each handed me a dime and said, "Call God." Then they spent the rest of the evening shaking their heads at me and consoling fucking Amy Hartnett on how her well-intentioned charity work had backfired.

The next morning when the charter bus pulled up to take us to the slopes, the bus driver, oblivious to the drama of the night before, approached the head counselor with a Hello Kitty purse containing two hundred dollars that he'd found on the floor of the bus. The counselor discreetly returned the purse to Amy without informing the other kids of what had really happened. The two of them let everybody believe that I was a thief and neither one ever offered me an apology. I suppose they hadn't had the sermon yet about the evils of being bigoted, Bible-thumping assholes.

Amy was never a true friend and I didn't miss her company or feel wounded by her actions; I felt enlightened. But Andrea and I had been close as sisters and her words were painful. The last thing she'd said to me was that I was a "tragic pawn of The Man." She pitied me in my self-loathing ignorance and added me to her list of "educated" black women who'd been successfully brainwashed by white society. I changed the outgoing message on my answering machine to say, "Hello, you've reached Uncle Tom. If you're The Man, there is no need to leave a message, I've already got it." She never rang me and the only person who heard it was somebody calling me for a job interview. That person reconsidered.

I never expected to hear from Andrea again, but when years later I got an insane message of garbled words ending with booming, riotous laughter, I knew exactly who it was and was thrilled. It wasn't happiness thrill, but that thrill gangbangers must feel before they rumble. My impulse was to call her back and tell her to fuckily shove that olive branch up her ass.

Obviously, she had heard that I was sick. She thought I was dying and wanted to take the autographed headshot of Rob Lowe from *The Outsiders*. It was signed to us both, but I'd bogarted it since 1983, refusing to let her take it home for fear that her crazy-ass brother would destroy it in some sadistic display of power. More than that, I just wanted it for myself. I wanted to gaze lustily at Soda Pop's hairless chest and soft, feminine features at my leisure. Andrea's sudden resurfacing was a worse harbinger than all the tests and studies combined. I was really going to die. Why else would she finally come forward?

It turned out that an e-mail about me was circulating. Some people simply deleted it and went on with their days, while others felt it was rude not to make contact of some sort. For a few, like Andrea, it was finally the excuse they needed to forgive me for the myriad of perceived offenses I'd committed. And being drugged was the perfect excuse for me to forgive my friends for their poor sportsmanship. Nothing wipes a slate clean faster than being diagnosed with a terminal disease. This was one of the best things about cancer.

chapter twelve

The second I started chemo my distress waned, but everybody else's waxed. As far as I was concerned, everything that could be done was being done to treat the disease. For everybody else, I became an official "cancer patient." Somebody was always staring at me, supporting me, dropping by to keep me company. I hardly had any time to myself. If I stayed in the bathroom for more than two minutes, Thibault would knock on the door and ask if I was okay. "I'm just hiding from all the f-ing people!" I wanted to scream. "I'm hiding in the toilet because it's the last place I get to go all by myself!"

In just two short, interminably long weeks I'd gone from the expatriate housewife life of virtual isolation, to being constantly supervised like a mental patient on suicide watch. People's intentions were noble, but their presence forced me to contemplate the reason for their visits. I had the most aggressive and lethal form of breast cancer and was probably going to die from it. It was an unpleasant truth, but one more easily forgotten while being ignored by my friends and family as I had been in France for so many months. I needed to find somewhere for my little family to be where we could have some semblance of normalcy and privacy.

My parents wanted us to stay with them, but I thought that if I was going to die of cancer, I'd rather not do it in a prison infirmary where I'd be serving my sentence for double homicide.

My parents are wonderful people, but the prospect of living with them again stressed me out. I imagined sexless months and restless nights, my sleep interrupted by my father's compulsive paper shredding and their five televisions blaring sports events and crime scene investigation shows.

My peace-loving mother, who wouldn't let us play with toy guns growing up and even banned us from watching the episode of *Little House on the Prairie* where Albert is accused of rape, watched hour after hour of gruesome murder mysteries. She merrily followed detectives searching for clues on the skinless female torso found floating in the river. Child poisonings and dwarf gang bangs were entertainment, but *The Dating Game, Who Wants to Marry a Millionaire?* and *Trading Spouses*—the things I wanted to watch—were degrading trash.

But more important than the promise of brawls over the remote control, my mother took her job as parent and hostess way too seriously. She'd spend all day taking care of us, fixing dinners, washing clothes. Having just started training a newly retired spouse, it was unfair to add the extra burden of our little family to her life.

Anyway, my one-and-only experience as a long-term guest turned out badly. I'm not sure if my presence caused this woman to become insane, or if she was already nuts. Billy was a friend of mine from college and Leah, his girlfriend, was one of those kooky L.A. chicks with an uninhibited sexuality that could only come from abuse. She was an issue hoarder, suffering from the typical eating disorders you expect in Los Angeles, plus bizarrely incestuous sibling rivalry and inappropriate parental relationships involving controlled substances. She'd say things like "This coke my dad gave me makes me want new tits" and "My sister's boyfriend never used condoms with me." These were statements to which Billy had grown accustomed, and made me wish I had money for my own apartment.

After two months of my sleeping on their couch, Billy and I were chummier than ever and Leah had had enough. She grew angrier and angrier, clues a self-respecting houseguest might pick up on, but since she took it out on Billy I didn't have to acknowledge that I was the problem. She raged at him, called him names, threatened to leave, and once even ordered Billy—not me, mind you—to get out.

Billy and I ignored her fuming and continued to clip supermarket circulars and prepare for our weekly trip to Ralph's for double coupon day. We'd gotten so good at manipulating the system, the real gift of an Ivy League education, that Ralph's was practically paying us to take the food. We once got a whole cart of groceries for $6.25. Granted, most items were things we never wanted and would only use reluctantly, but it was free, 1992, and we were victims of a recession.

As we were getting in the car Leah shrieked, "Don't forget my tampons! I've been wearing this same pad for two days," at which I shuddered and Billy said, "Like that smell wasn't all the headline we needed." But we didn't have a tampax coupon so Leah didn't get her feminine hygiene products. When she looked through the paper bags and found three cans of asparagus spears, all dented, a box of matzo, and six bags of tortillas, I thought she'd scream. Instead she stood behind Billy as he lay on the sofa watching *Northern Exposure*, pulled her pants down, tore her supersaturated maxi-pad from her dingy underpants, and stuck it, adhesive side down, to the top of Billy's head. He ripped it off and without even turning around to aim, flung it back at her. It landed on the flat surface where her future breast implants would go. Suddenly, she had made herself clear. The houseguest had overstayed her welcome.

In college I thought my parents' house had burned down. One cool fall New York day, while studying for midterms, I got a call from my mom. This in itself was highly unusual because she hated making long-distance calls. She lived in constant fear of phone bills. When forced to make a long-distance call, she talked superfast and rushed to hang up.

My mother asked if I'd been watching television. I told her no, that I was studying, which sounded like a lie but in this case was actually true. When she suggested that I put down my books and turn on the television while she waited, I knew something was terribly wrong. I explained that the television was in the lounge. I would have to walk down the hall, find the news, watch it, and then walk all the way back to my room. That could mean a minute or more of dead, wasted phone time. She insisted.

In the lounge I found a room full of people staring blankly at a shot of my parents' California neighborhood in flames. Eucalyptus trees burned like torches. Houses exploded. People were being held back by barricades, crying and attempting to break past police. Fire trucks were leaving the scene because the pumps, after three days of hosing off everything in sight, had drained the reservoir.

I rushed back to the phone, only to discover that my mother had already hung up. She just couldn't handle that open line stretching from coast to coast, twenty cents, forty cents, sixty cents extra on the phone bill.

I had no idea where they were, or if everyone was safe. Had they managed to rescue the photo albums or the cat? That night I dreamed of the flames spreading through my house, licking and then ravenously swallowing my love letters from Maceo. I could see the red silk ribbon I'd tied them up with curl, melt, and turn to ash. I imagined the portrait I'd done of my father when I was eight. He was jogging through a park and had on two-toned shorts and a big Scorpio medallion. It hung on the wood-paneled wall of his study, right above his beloved shredder. Now the construction paper was turning black and his big toothy grin was disappearing into the flames. My whole childhood was carbonizing.

The television showed a neighborhood that looked like a bombed-out Beirut with nothing left but a landscape of rubble and forests of chimney stacks. It was three days before I found out our house was one of only a handful that had survived the firestorm.

Now, years later, I lay in my sister's bed, my mind occupied not with dying or orphaning my son, or being disfigured, but with obsessive nightmares about losing my home again, my stupid apartment in Paris I'd only lived in for three months. In my dreams things kept disappearing off the counters. First my candlesticks, then the napkin rings. I opened drawers and they were empty. In one dream the big iron key to the front lock wouldn't work. When I peered through the keyhole, a huge nipple eyeball blinked back at me; it had locked me out of my own life. I woke up knowing that I'd never feel any sort of peace until I found someplace to be.

Rebecca's mom, Karen, had a little cottage behind her house that she meant to use someday as a design studio. It had only one room but was furnished and newly renovated. Her estate had a pool, tennis court, and playground for Lucas. There was a garden and greenhouse begging for attention. When I called her up crying, she didn't hesitate to offer it to us, rent-free, for as long as we needed it. She even said she wanted the company, that we were doing her a service. Truth or lie, it was exactly what I needed to hear. I felt like we'd been rescued, like this whole debacle was suddenly manageable.

So after moving his wife and son, our one suitcase, and a new IKEA bed into the cottage, Thibault went back to Paris, packed up all our freshly unpacked things, and put them in storage. He notified his clients; I quit my job, in a blubbery, hysterical, one-sided phone call. And three weeks after leaving France for a quick visit to California we were the three newest residents of the sleepy, semirural postcard that is Sonoma County.

chapter thirteen

It only took about a month of baldness before I started thinking that having hair was symptomatic of some sort of mental disorder. It was equivalent to wearing sunglasses at night or shaving off your eyebrows and then painting them on in hopeful expressions. I stared at everybody's hair, but especially the hair of people with blow-dried bangs, the kind that curl under and look parched. Nothing could make me understand what that dead fiber was on people's heads, other than a disgusting, filthy and absurdly time-consuming affectation.

My own head was no longer the mottled dome I exposed that first day. Now it was brown forehead all the way back to my neck, no stubble, just smooth, rubbery skin stretched tight and waxy. It looked magnificent and I spent hours caressing it. Covering it with a wig would have been the epitome of absurd. The synthetic ones felt like wearing big wax lips over my own; and the real-hair ones felt like an appendix transplant in the process of being rejected. Baldness was comfortable for me.

It soon became clear, though, that wearing a wig wasn't always about my own comfort. My bald head was like the elephant in the room. People had a hard time acting normal around me when I was bald. They tended to move slowly, as if quick motion might reactivate tumor growth, and they spoke carefully, often whispering and avoiding certain words.

I felt like the whole world had gone mad. My friend Frederika flew across the country to spend six hours naming every goddamned plant in my garden. Then she wrote me an unbearably long and poetic note about the fig tree and sunset colors. There weren't even any meaningful allusions or insightful metaphors to make decrypting her horrendous handwriting worthwhile.

It took several odd visits that seemed to start off normal and quickly deteriorated to realize the problem was twofold. One, people are naturally cautious around illness and need safe subjects; and two, "chemo brain" had left me with the cognitive and analytical skills of a small rodent. I was stupider than ever.

People tried to talk to me like an adult, but couldn't. At the peak of my imbecility, Thibault said he was going to cut the squash in quarters and I actually argued with him, saying, "But we need four pieces! Four! What will we do with quarters?" He looked heartbroken.

When we first met, I was an engineering student who had developed her own ingenious version of calculus. It was longer and more complicated than the standard Newtonian and Leibniz versions, often taking hours to solve the most basic equations, but it functioned (get it?) nonetheless. To date, my not equating quarters with the number four may have been my unsexiest moment. At least until my upcoming mastectomy.

I also learned that death-threatening disease, as advertised by baldness, attracts lunatics. Weirdos wanted to touch me, touch my head, and pet my arms like I was some kind of dog. But it was only the oddest, most marginalized people who found the courage to approach me. I felt like a cast member from *Star Trek: Enterprise*. Once I was on the street just talking to some friends when I sensed this presence behind me. The pores on my neck flexed, forgetting there was no hair to stand on end. I turned around to find this braless, middle-aged woman with huge blue eyes focused intently on my forehead.

Her arm reached out and rested on my shoulder. Then she snatched it back as if it were a child wandering into traffic. "I know," she said, "how to heal you, if you like, I mean, if you believe." I just looked at her. "I healed a cat once, it had leukemia." She whispered the leukemia part. Perhaps she'd been an old Jewish woman before she became New Age. "Just let me know, no pressure." She continued to stare at my head, apparently waiting for an answer.

"But I'm allergic to cats. Does that matter?" She confused my confusion with mocking and shrank back. I hadn't meant to sound disingenuous. "No, seriously, does it matter?" She excused herself and backed away, leaving me feeling as though I was the crazy one.

In addition to hippies, I realized I could also do without my fingernails. About midway through the chemo my nails started to change color. Starting at the base of the nail bed, near the little moons, purplish bruises appeared, first on my thumb, then on my index finger, and slowly spread toward my pinkie. My fingernails were so sensitive that I found myself lifting things with the heel of my palm and turning pages with my elbows. Slowly, the purple crept higher and higher up my nail bed and the white slowly pulled back to meet it. After a few weeks the only thing holding my nails on at all was the overgrown cuticle. It was ugly and I hid my hands in my pockets, or inside extra long sleeves to avoid being spotted.

My palms also started to turn a dark purplish black. They looked as though I'd forgotten to wear gloves while dying hair. I washed them compulsively, but the stain was coming from the inside. One of my chemo drugs was also a dye. In addition to killing fast-growing cells, it also managed to color slow-growing ones such as palm skin. I was convinced that I was finally being punished for my most racist thought ever.

When I first moved to France I couldn't understand anything. I watched television for practice and tried to piece together story lines. One afternoon, as I sat in the apartment alone, a news story came on. On the screen was a white couple dressed in khakis, holding the two ugliest black newborns I had ever seen. These children were black—not brown, but black, with silky little pompadours and big white diapers. They had round brown eyes that rolled around their scrunched-up little faces and they grasped the white couple's fingers and clothing with a strength and dexterity I found quite advanced for their apparent age.

I simply could not understand what the reporter was saying, who this couple was, or what part of deepest Africa these ugly children came from. Nor could I comprehend why these children would be subjected to a press conference and all those flashing lights, screaming journalists, and germs. I understood that the babies were twins and here in Paris. They couldn't possibly be on the news because they were the ugliest children ever born. At least, I thought, they had each other so as not to have to face this cruel world alone. Luckily, Thibault came home to explain what was happening. He listened for a moment and reported that twin gorillas had just been born at the Paris zoo.

Now it was coming back to haunt me. My palms and fingernails were slowly turning black, like those ugly little gorillas. I was just like the evil temptress in that movie from the '30s, *Freaks,* who gets transformed into a legless chicken as punishment for vanity and cruelty. Thankfully, over several months, my nails restored themselves and eventually appeared normal. I remain convinced that my recovery was due to my heartfelt and sincere prayers for forgiveness to all the ugly black children and apes worldwide.

About the same time my fingernails fell off I switched chemotherapy drugs, from Adriamycin/Cytoxin to Taxol. The A/C combination was very strong but I handled it well and suffered none of the really uncomfortable side effects. The Taxol was different. I had an allergic reaction that lasted for weeks. About two days after the drug was first administered I developed a head-to-toe rash. It started on my fingers and toes and slowly crept toward my torso. After about five days I itched all over like I had scabies, which I'd not had at that point but would experience once Lucas started preschool. Knowing not to scratch, I sought relief by slapping myself. I slapped my arms and thighs, the harder, the better. I started using a wooden spoon, but it was leaving welt marks that actually intensified the itching as they disappeared.

Then I started rubbing, first with my palm. That didn't

work because my palms were covered with the rash as well, and touching them just made it itch more. So I wrapped a sock around my wooden spoon and tried to rub myself with that. Early on, when I could still exhibit restraint, it did provide some relief. But I soon lost control and started to rub feverishly until the top layer of my skin was gone. At that point I was so itchy I just gave up and started scratching with my fingernail stumps. This caused extreme pain, as my naked fingertips were hypersensitive. I itched everywhere: the soles of my feet, back of my neck, armpits, chest, elbows. I couldn't quench it and became so frustrated that I curled into a ball and cried.

All day long I slathered myself in hydrocortisone creams, gels, and sprays. I took Benadryl, anti-inflammatories, and painkillers. Nothing helped. At night the itching kept me awake. I tried meditation, repeating the mantra, "Not itchy. Not itchy." On weekends I went to my sister's house and lay prostrate on her abrasive shag carpet in my bra and underwear. I'd writhe around like an eel in heat until the rug burns were more painful than the itching. Then I meditated until the burning passed and I could writhe around again.

It was during one of these rug sessions—although this time I was in my own home, curled onto a sisal doormat, without bra or panties, and had added the sock-dressed-spoon slapping action—that I realized this scenario of a naked, hairless woman abrading herself with a carpet and kitchen utensils, roiling and moaning animatedly on the floor was Meredith. It was also the moment my friends peered in the window hoping to find me ready to leave for lunch. They knocked politely and mouthed that they'd wait in the car. We all passed the remainder of the day pretending nobody had seen me compromised and my mental health was peachy.

Not everyone, however, was so kind or forgiving. Travis is the kind of guy who on a road trip will stop to pick wildflowers because he needs a break from crying over an audio version of *The Secret Life of Bees*. Then he'll drive some more, roll into a country store, and buy canned beer, porn, and ammo. He went to Burning Man wearing a homemade goat-pelt vest, cowboy hat, and necklace of teeth that he himself had extracted from a personal boar kill. Burning Man, he explained, was all about radical self-expression manifesting in the form of toplessness: "There were naked girls everywhere, like a thousand tits on parade." I told him I wanted to go next year and he said, "Then there'll be like a thousand and one tits on parade!"

"Who?"

"Forget it, Meredith. I think you have cancer between your ears."

My sister, Angela, only treated me with kid gloves to the extent that she changed her typical "Shut up" to "I'm going to beat your ass when you're better." She didn't completely avoid the topic of mortality, either, which was wildly refreshing. One evening at dinner everyone in my family was yelling at one another across the table, repeating themselves endlessly and gesturing flamboyantly. It was not out of anger that these theatrics emerged, but because deafness runs on both sides and wearing hearing aids does not.

My brother argued that nobody could eat six saltine crackers in one minute.

"How could anybody still be hungry after all the food I fixed?" my mother asked.

"It's just a challenge. I'll bet anybody twenty bucks."

"Now we have to pay you to eat crackers? I paid for twenty-one years of tuition between the three of you. No, twenty-four! I'm not paying twenty cents to watch you eat anything." This was my father, of course.

"No, I'll pay you twenty dollars," said Douglas.

"What am I going to do with your twenty dollars? Retire? Save it and buy some decent socks."

Angela leaned toward me and said in a normal voice, but for practical purposes a whisper, "Please don't die and leave me alone with these people."

chapter fourteen

When I was twenty-five I went to the family reunion in St. Augustine, Florida. St. Augustine is the oldest continually inhabited city in the United States and unfortunately reflects the nation's sordid history. There is a Spanish fort, complete with a moat, the marker indicating the site of the Apalachee Indian massacre, and, right in the middle of the town, the old slave market that tour guides point out excitedly, like I'm going to jump out of my seat and take a picture of that depraved shit. My family has lived in or around St. Augustine for hundreds of years. A few of us surely passed through that open-air building, and we weren't on vacation.

This vacation's traveling party included my dad and his brother, Edward, my cousins Kathy and Johnny, my sister, Angela, her three-year-old daughter, Kendall, and me. My brother stayed home working as a summer associate in a law firm, and my mother pretended she didn't hear my father when he invited her to come.

My dad and uncle are only two years apart and were very close growing up. They had the same friends, went to the same schools, and, until my uncle left for college, slept every night in the same room. They look and sound so much alike that growing up people masked their confusion by asking, "Hey, Norton, how's your brother?" But superficialities aside, nobody really listening would ever confuse the two.

My uncle is extremely present. He is also accessible in a way my father is not. And he swears in front of the children, something my father would NEVER do, and we'd never do around him. (Although he did once call Ronald Reagan a jackass.)

Even though they lived on opposite coasts for almost forty years, it only took seconds for them to slip into their old patterns. When we arrived in St. Augustine, the first thing we did was rent a minivan and go visit Mrs. Gordon, the schoolteacher. She was almost a hundred years old, maybe two hundred, and had been a friend of my grandparents from before they'd had kids, like in the early 1930s. My dad and uncle started arguing in the car about the quickest route to her house, a house neither of them had been to since the summer of 1947.

"John, you need to turn left here."

"You don't even drive, Edward."

"But I can see. I pay attention."

"Are you saying I don't pay attention?"

"I thought we were talking about me?"

"I remember distinctly, we go straight."

This was forty seconds into the ride. Meanwhile the air-conditioning wasn't working and it was 102 degrees outside, with 90 percent humidity. A mysterious alarm, the source of which we never found, kept going *Ping!Ping!Ping!* like submarine radar in my claustrophobic sister's ear. The back windows didn't roll down, but popped out about three inches and Angela had her nose flush to the glass, trying not to hyperventilate. Kendall, who rarely spoke to anyone, decided to practice knock knock jokes on Johnny, who seemed perpetually disgusted even in the best settings, but even more so by the inanity of her jokes. And Kathy, having fairly severe Down syndrome, moaned and rocked in the rear seat.

When we did get to Mrs. Gordon's house, which *had* been to the left and we *had* missed the turn, thirty heat-stroking minutes later, the tiniest woman in the world answered the door. She had on white polyester slacks and a pink wool sweater and tiny children's pink ballet slippers. I blinked hard trying to figure out if she was real or not. Luckily she didn't see me gawking because, from her vantage point of about four feet, she was looking down, as if expecting to greet a child. When all she saw were two pairs of old sweaty knees, her eyes shot up, her hands shot to her cheeks in astonishment, and she cried, "Why, Edward, John, you are grown men!"

The two men that stood before her were gray and mustachioed, one of them holding his granddaughter's pink vinyl backpack. Mrs. Gordon's eyes lingered on it for a moment, probably wondering if it was his. But they both still had the huge toothy grins and the good posture of boys raised right. They kissed her simultaneously on opposite cheeks, handed her flowers, and introduced the brood behind them.

Kendall couldn't contain her glee. The house was pink. The walls, carpet, tiles, cabinets, furniture, toilet, drapes, all pink. Mrs. Gordon even served us pink lemonade out of pink frosted glasses. She told us about the last time she had a real heart-to-heart with our grandmother, twenty years dead. This was long before that, even, before she'd moved away from St. Augustine. My grandmother told Mrs. Gordon that she was going to New York to be with John Norton and be a seamstress. Mrs. Gordon asked her if John knew she was coming, because nobody had heard from him for a while, and my grandmother bristled. "But it was true!" said Mrs. Gordon. "When John left St. Augustine no one noticed him looking back." She remembered all the names of all the people in all the pictures around her house. She even remembered our names from the second we walked in the door. (I, however, had to call all my cousins at the reunion "Cousin.") She was still involved in the community and very active. In fact, she'd just shot a national commercial for an insurance company where she wore a bathing suit and water-skied! She said it just like that, with an exclamation point.

When we left she gave the kids—kids meaning anyone un-der fifty—a piece of strawberry candy. Then she reached way up and patted my dad and uncle on their heads. "Why, you are balding, Edward!" Before my uncle could say anything she closed the screen door and told them to "be good boys and don't cause any trouble." They nodded obediently and climbed back into the van.

Within seconds the two old men were complaining: "How come we didn't get any candy?" My sister put a stop to it, say-ing, "You just promised not to cause any trouble!"

Afterward we went to meet the rest of our family. When we got to the park I approached the wrong bunch of picnicking black people and had be steered in the right direction by my sister. She had some memory of these folks, having been born on the East Coast and spending a few years among them. Some of them I had never met, and others I had seen only a handful of times in my whole life. It could have been anybody's family.

I sat next to Kathy on the picnic table bench and she held on to my arm, rocking. I wondered if she remembered who I was, that I used to be small and we would wrap our legs around each other on the Sit'n Spin. Then she pointed to a statue nearby and murmured, "Grandma, Grandma." I knew instantly what she was talking about.

When my grandmother Blanche died, in January 1981, we went back to New York without winter coats. My sister might have had one, but my brother, Douglas, only had layered sweaters, and I only had a brown and tan polyester-fill vest. In California, you might need a jacket in the morning, but by noon, even in winter, it is warm enough to do without. Consequently, kids were forever losing their coats, and other parents were forever replacing them. Eloise Norton had decided she wasn't replacing another lost jacket for my brother or me. It didn't matter that we were going to New York in the dead of winter, when the mercury topped off at 9 degrees Fahrenheit. We ran from the car to the church, stunned by the cold, and from the church to the reception hall with frozen tears in our eyes. Luckily, my mother didn't force us to go to the cemetery; we might have gotten hypothermia or been taken into custody by Child Protective Services.

At our grandmother's funeral Kathy was really upset. They were close and Kathy couldn't seem to understand why Grandma wouldn't wake up. I remember standing next to Kathy at the casket, looking at our Blanche in a wig we'd never seen, and wondering, just like my mentally retarded cousin, why she wouldn't wake up. We looked closely to see if she was breathing or twitching, or wiggling at all. But she was as still as a statue. I held on to Kathy's arm and, when nobody was looking, nudged my grandmother's hand. It was cold and stone hard.

The biggest event of our trip to St. Augustine was not the reunion, but visiting the mythical alligator farm that had emotionally scarred both my dad and uncle as children. Nobody is quite sure what, exactly, happened there on a sunny afternoon in 1943, but it certainly had a greater impact on these two boys than the world war raging in Europe. Nowadays the farm is called a zoological park and has a gift shop and railings. When the brothers were six and eight, it was apparently an open pit of writhing reptiles, clawing at one another on the muddy slopes for tasty hunks of skinny boy asses.

My father has joked about alligators for as long as I can remember, covering his eyes and cringing when they appeared on television, and even leaving the *National Geographic* issues spotlighting the creatures unopened. He checked the park hours twice before we got in the van, and then called back a third time to see if we needed a reservation. Each time they were open with plenty of availability he looked disappointed.

My uncle claimed that he didn't need to go to any alligator park, face any demons, because that park wasn't where he'd been traumatized. He remembered distinctly, something both he and my father say often, that he wasn't afraid of them until the dock incident at the grandparents' house. He'd been warned a hundred times if once to stay out of that marsh; it was teeming with gators. It was probably just a scare tactic employed to keep him dry, because when he did fall in, not ten minutes after arriving, nothing ate him. No one screamed, or at least not loud enough to be heard over Edward's own screaming. Someone just reached down and pulled him out, all forty soaking-wet, panic-stricken pounds of him. The fact is that any alligators in the water could have easily walked the hundred feet right up the banks, across the narrow road, straight into the family's yard. Nobody had warned him to stay out of the yard then, and fifty years later, in that same yard, he seemed perfectly relaxed eating crab and hard-boiled eggs.

He outright refused, however, to enter the alligator farm, preferring to sit in the parking lot with Kathy, who looked perfectly serene, even sedate, but, Edward assured us, was already riled up and on the verge of a very dramatic outburst. Johnny's habitual look of disgust seemed more ingrained than ever as he shook his head at his father and took the ticket handed to him.

My father was surprisingly gung ho, probably from feeling superior to his brother, and marched through the turnstile confidently. Once inside, though, he lingered by the fence farthest from the pit. Slowly, he inched forward. After a few minutes he stood right at the edge of the deck hanging over the lagoon and gleefully watched the gator wrestler toss nutria carcasses, skulls intact with big orange teeth, at the animals. They swarmed all over one another like enormous black maggots, chomping and swallowing whole whatever they caught.

We followed him over the series of low wooden bridges that made the nature trail. It cleared the green algae that covered the lagoon by about two feet and rattled and bounced in a disconcerting way. Spots of scaly nostrils and prehistoric eyelids were all you could see of the seemingly hundreds of creatures lurking below. My father stayed far behind the man so fat his Bermuda shorts rose up between his thighs, revealing chafed red patches; he wouldn't share the bowing span of bridge with that fat man.

I spent most of my time watching my father flirt with courage. He let his foot hang slightly over the bridge, then, realizing it was there, forced himself to leave it . . . but only for ten seconds before he reeled it in. He even turned his back to the pond and posed nonchalantly long enough for me to take his picture, but chalantly spun back around the second the shutter clicked.

When we finally left, after an hour or so, my father moseyed over to the minivan. Uncle Edward's arms were crossed defensively. "I thought you'd only be gone a few minutes. Kathy's losing it. She really needs to get back to the hotel." Kathy was standing in the shade of a tree lazily tracing circles in the sand with a palm frond.

The night before we left there was a big family banquet with everyone present. People spoke and toasted, we took pictures by generation, and then there was a talent show. Cousin started to sing, off note and off beat. Then Other Cousin danced with the grace of a Russian bear. And Cousin with Overcoiffed Hair recited a poem with profound structural problems. I could not have been more entertained, or felt a greater sense of family . . . until I realized nobody had told me about this ahead of time, or asked if I wanted to perform. And they hadn't done it for the exact same reason that I'd approached the wrong people in the park when we first arrived; there was nothing connecting us but the shared, stereotype-shattering gene that made us book-smart but talentless performers. My family were the people sitting at the table, the ones who knew to properly arrange the vowels in my names and dismissed my pouting by saying, "How are you insulted when you don't even have a talent to perform?"

chapter fifteen

Almost a decade later, faced with the very real prospect of leaving my son motherless, I remembered that reunion. If I died Thibault would take Lucas back to France and my family would probably see him once every five years during these really strained visits that took Lucas away from his friends and ruined his summer vacations. He'd grow up French and white. Maybe as a teenager he'd start listening to West Coast/Oakland rap and think he was getting in touch with his roots, but really he'd have no idea how far off target that was. The family that spawned and raised his own mother would feel as irrelevant to him as that banquet hall of second cousins felt to me.

Eight weeks into chemotherapy I saw a therapist at a friend's insistence. I was visiting Wah, my college roommate, in Los Angeles where she had scheduled two full days of activities for me, the last of which was to visit a "spiritual adviser." I thought he was going to read tarot cards and tea leaves or something, but within thirty seconds of sitting across from him gazing at me serenely, I deduced that he was, in fact, a psychologist, not a psychic. His shelves were covered with books about Freud and Jung. There was no jewel-colored satin or velvet in sight, and the only crystal ball was a Murano glass paperweight placed artistically on his desk.

We discussed me for about fifteen minutes. Then I ranted

about Lance Armstrong for another fifteen. He wasn't surprised at all that I wanted to poke a stick in Lance's spokes. I asked him if he thought I needed a therapist. He said no, not on the subject of my cancer; I seemed very much in touch with my feelings. He suspected that my friends and family simply confused my coping well with being in denial. I certainly did not need to fake a breakdown for their benefit. Then he said the worst thing anybody had said to me so far. He said that children orphaned before eight years old can't remember their parents. He suggested that I make videos for Lucas to remember me by.

I appreciated his frankness and considered the videos a good idea. He was one of the few people who had spoken to me as though his words were not rocks and I was not glass. But by the next day, I was obsessed with the vision of myself rotting in the cold earth while Lucas watched a tape of me teaching him how to tie his shoes or drive a stick shift. These were things he'd probably never even need in the Velcro-and-electric-car future that loomed ahead. I'd be hairless and dressed in the future's equivalent of a leisure suit, giving him advice that had probably long since been proven wrong. It would be like in *Sleeper* when the future doctor offers Woody Allen a cigarette and he declines, saying he doesn't smoke. The doctor replies, "But why? It's the best thing for you!" I'd be telling Lucas to wear sunscreen or not eat too much bacon and look like an ignoramus. Instead of his not recollecting me at all, he'd remember me as an unstylish source of misinformation.

Plus, I'd done a really good job of not fixating on leaving my son motherless. I had moments, of course, when I didn't want to get pricked once again for a blood test or infusion, when all I wanted in the world was smothered fried chicken and syrup-drenched waffles, then I purposely conjured the image of my abandoning Lucas. It served as motivation to make me do whatever unpleasant thing needed to be done, or not to do something bad. But it wasn't an image I dwelled upon. A two-second glimpse was all that was necessary to make me put down the waffle or relax my hand so the phlebotomist could find a vein. Anything longer would reduce me to tears.

But what the therapist said was true: if I died prematurely Lucas wouldn't even have any context in which to place me. There would be no me, no memory of me, and no reliable sources from which to conjure up an image of me. Thibault's commitment to me aside, I'd only known the man for three years, and much of that time was spent with a major communication problem.

People need their mothers. They certainly need them when they are one and eight and fifteen. Maybe by forty having a mother is a luxury and technically, although you may enjoy her company, you are sufficiently equipped for life.

People who lose their mothers young have a hard time being happy. Contentment eludes them. My friend Shirin suddenly lost her mother when she was seventeen. She spent her twenties trying not to grasp on to anyone for fear that they would just disappear on their way out to vacuum the car. Her life motto became "Better to walk on bare floors than have the rug pulled out from under you." I doubt she saw her mother's death as a betrayal, but it certainly planted seeds of mistrust, and she was well over eight years old.

Would Lucas' life be ruined? Would he be an emotional midget or worse, a damaged monster? It was not as if he wouldn't still have a father and four grandparents, three great-grandmothers, five uncles, and two aunts. There would be people to love him. My sister alone would provide him with all the kisses his smooth little cheeks could stand. Were auntie-kisses enough?

Maybe Thibault would remarry and his new wife would fully embrace little Lucas, raising him as her own. I just seriously doubted that happening. Thibault barely got together with me. Contrary to the great French lover myth, Thibault has no moves and reads no signs. I had to throw myself at him shamelessly for months before he realized I was interested, and even then he was so shy I had to get him drunk. Of course, since he drinks all the time and I drink rarely, the drunk one ended up being me. Luckily, my intoxicated stumbling landed me right on top of him with my lips close enough to his that he only had to pucker and we made contact. If not for that, he'd still be single, staying up all night in game rooms battling cyber enemies. Consequently, I was not putting my hopes into Thibault's finding another wife as a replacement mama for my baby.

But even though I said I would take the psychologist's advice to make the tapes, and meant it when I spoke, I knew it would never happen. Making the tapes would ensure my early death. If I made the tapes, Lucas would learn me from them.

Who ever heard of some old lady organizing the attic and coming across a box of tapes, saying, "Oh my gosh, sonny boy, remember when we thought I was going to die and we made these?" Then the family pops them into the player and spends an evening laughing over the archaic appliances in the background.

Furthermore, it was doubtful that I could accurately represent myself during the tapings. I wasn't exactly the witty beauty my friends and family had grown to love. This was partially due to a drug called G-CSF, short for granulocyte colony-stimulating factor, an immunobooster that increased production of blood cells to counteract the suppression caused by the chemotherapy. One of the side effects of G-CSF is what a casual observer might describe as intense rage and hatred toward all things living and dead. It is as though the drug were designed to fuel the global war machine. With me, perfectly innocuous situations were elevated to the intolerable. People's good intentions were twisted and mangled until they warranted venomous attacks. It was all but impossible to harness my rage.

It got to the point where I dreaded taking the injections. Not that I was eager at the beginning, but I washed my hands, prepared the syringe, cleaned a small patch of skin on my chubby lower abdomen, and punctured my belly with the control of a professional nurse. After several weeks, however, my belly was bruised and sensitive. I couldn't stab myself. I just held the needle tip against my stomach and applied slow, steady pressure. The syringe formed a deep indentation before finally breaking through the skin and sinking unresisted into the subcutaneous fat. It was like poking a chopstick through a hot water bottle filled with warm custard. Sometimes it took twenty minutes. But more of a deterrent than the pain was the knowledge that within half an hour rage would start to rise in me like feculent water in a backed-up toilet.

There were certain chores I was too irritable to do, like going to Wal-Mart. It was too messy. The shelves were disordered, the lighting poor. The little Wal-Mart price slash signs were all askew. After ten minutes I'd kick open the front door, gasp for air, and scream, "How can you people bear it? Aaaaaah!"

I tried to restrict my outbursts to inanimate objects and strangers, but sometimes lacked the control. During those periods I did my best to avoid friends, family, and valuables. This was not easy, due to the fact that I had an almost constant entourage of well-wishers supporting me. I was sometimes abusive and had homicidal thoughts.

I explained my temper issues to everyone. They had the choice to remain in my company or retreat to a safe distance. Thibault was perhaps the one exception. Being that he was my husband and we lived together in a one-room house, he was forced to remain in my presence at times when I knew he must have wanted to be elsewhere.

He suffered much undeserved punishment. Some nights I kicked him simply because he was sleeping so soundly. Other times I shrieked, threw my plate, and dramatically slammed the door because I could see his tongue. I could not tolerate a wrinkled collar or smudges on his glasses. It didn't matter that our iron was in storage and Lucas found it hilarious to pull the glasses off his face whenever they were within reach. But Thibault never returned the insults, not once. He just waited until I quieted down, gave me a hug, and said to himself more than to me, "Just two more days until the injections are done. It's not you, it's the medicine, *chérie*." I know he wanted to hold a pillow over my face and suffocate me. And nobody would have blamed him, except me. I would have fought him like a rabid, cornered wolverine.

The first half of the two-week chemo cycle was mental torture, the second week, physical. Once the medicine started to take effect and increase the production of blood cells, my bones would ache from the strain on my bone marrow. The thing about the aching was that it didn't radiate from the usual places, namely the joints. Everybody understands a sore knee or shoulder, a strained ankle or twisted elbow. Pain from mid-femur is unsettling. It felt as though my thighbone was being stretched lengthwise. Eventually, if the stretching didn't stop, the bone would tear—not snap, but tear. The pain was not acute, but perpetual pressure that left me feeling confused and walking awkwardly.

I measured my height four times a day. If my bones really were stretching, then surely I must be getting taller. Thibault humored me, thickening the same black line on the doorjamb. He never once poked me between the eyebrows and spat, "Are you stupid? Stupid?" which is what I did to him when he forgot the sixty-seven new cable station channel numbers. No, he just looked perplexed and exclaimed, "Well, you certainly look taller!" It was so sweet I vowed to start faking orgasms, just as soon as I got the chance.

When I was five or six my family flew back east from California several times. I used to love sitting by the window and watching the plane rise above the cottony clouds. I wished I had a glass jar to put some clouds in so I could take them home. But whenever we were packing, I would forget to put the jar in my red Starsky and Hutch backpack with the white Ford Torino stripe. By the time we got to cruising altitude, I was totally heartbroken at my missed opportunity and put Fruit Stripes chewing gum in my own hair as some sort of six-year-old's version of self-flagellation.

Every time I forgot my cloud jar, my mother would offer other solutions. I could use a Styrofoam coffee cup, or a barf bag. She even offered her own Louis Vuitton purse, but it was so packed with receipts and Cornsilk face powder that my clouds, once I got them, would look filthy and littered. There was simply no solution besides the glass jar. She sat me on her lap, fished the gum out of my hair, and promised to help me remember the jar next time.

Thibault was capable of loving me as purely as a parent loves a child. It was unconditional and without malice. He never wanted me to suffer, even when I deserved it, even when I begged for it. And he went to great lengths to protect me from disappointment. His ability to let me live in a world of fanciful perceptions and my own interpretations is exactly what I needed in a husband—a partner in life determined to not burst my bubble.

Maybe Thibault would be enough for my son if cancer claimed me. He could rub my lotion into Lucas' moist skin after his bath, so he'd remember my smell. He could tell my stories and bake my cupcakes. He could fill our son's childhood with enough glitter and atonal melodies that Lucas would absorb the essence of the woman he'd only envisage from pictures. Maybe the placid satisfaction, the embarrassing relief that my early death let me off the hook as far as ever having to accomplish anything, didn't have to feel so shameful.

chapter sixteen

My father described my cancer as the worst thing that ever happened to him and admitted that reading about my disease and treatment was the first time since studying for state medical boards forty years ago that he cried over a textbook.

I had to think about whether or not I believed that. My father was a maudlin man who miraculously managed to remain authoritative and masculine through his sniffling. He cried easily, often, and over an assortment of things: weddings, funerals, graduations, Olympic medal ceremonies, Church of Jesus Christ of Latter-day Saints commercials, a new paper shredder, anything. It seemed implausible that a textbook hadn't triggered his tears in nearly half a century.

I moved to France just a few weeks after September 11, 2001. I missed everyone in my family except my father. CNN provided constant reminders of him. Every few minutes of 9/11 coverage was punctuated with some typically hypermanly man, a fireman, policeman, or steelworker, choking back sobs while tears streamed down his cheeks and an American flag waved in the distance. The day before my departure I counted fourteen American flags on display in my parents' house.

Like America, my brother, sister, and I were an obvious source of pride for my father. But some of the same things that triggered tears of pride also triggered tears of disappointment. My crazed aimlessness, for example, was evidence of a sense of freedom he never imagined growing up as a black man in postrenaissance Harlem. He worked long and hard to provide me with everything I needed, from a stable home to private schools, tennis lessons, and plane tickets to Europe. He did all of this because he firmly believed I would make something of myself and give back to society. But rather than make good use of that freedom, I saw it as a means to indulge my most low-brow whims.

Most of my whims he simply ignored, but when I told him about wanting to live in an Airstream trailer he actually screamed and covered his ears. "The redneck trash would really love to see my daughter in the doublewide next door!" I tried to explain that doublewide trailers were a whole other aesthetic, but it fell on plugged ears. He hadn't worked like a mule for forty years so that his daughter could live in a house on wheels, or worse, one propped up on cinder blocks.

He had a certain sensitivity to housing issues so I refrained from telling him when I found a real live tree house to live in. Twenty-two-year-olds without college diplomas, or at least with diplomas in ecology or botany, could live in trees. His daughter needed a milled-wood habitation built with permits. This was not exactly the picture he'd had in his mind of my taking the world by the horns.

As far as tree houses go, this one was fairly luxurious. That is not to say it was insulated. It had running water and electricity, but no bathroom. The tree house hamleteers shared a toilet and shower close to the entrance of the property. There were five houses but only two others were occupied. One was lived in by the "developer," a Grizzly Adams–type hippie with muttonchop sideburns and an Abraham Lincoln beard. He wore a red-and-gray ski bib pretty much all the time and constantly rubbed his home-brewed organic beer belly. A girl who called herself Maple but whose mail was addressed to Jennifer occupied the other tree house. She didn't shave her legs or anything else and she marched about the property singing Ani DiFranco songs in cutoff bike shorts that showcased an overgrown fluorescent orange bush that matched her honky dreads. Her house was built at the base of a great oak tree, the mammoth trunk of which went right through her living room. Its gnarled roots, covered by filthy Persian carpets, warped her dirt floor. Bead curtains with images of the Madonna and Buddha were strung from the lowest branches to form makeshift walls. Hidden in every crevice of this driftwood and string tree house was a tiny, stuffed mouse dressed in a flamboyant costume.

Maple Jennifer had a problem with mice. They ran across the canyon floor and waltzed freely into her hobbit home. For months she battled them with steel wool and all sorts of humane traps. She had even, despite severe allergies, gotten a great big tomcat named Wiley. He was ironically killed by a coyote. She decided finally to take a more psychological approach and enrolled in a taxidermy class at the community college. With a minor investment in skinning knives, forceps, clay, wax, twine, preserving solutions, and tiny glass eyes, she was set to begin her deranged war against the rodents.

Her first challenge was to capture a few mice and prepare

the specimens. I expected her to fumble about and cry, but she was quite nimble, snatching them by the tails and cleanly snapping their necks. She then washed, traced, and skinned them, disjointed their limbs, and soaked the tiny pelts in alcohol. While they were curing, she fashioned artificial forms out of Styrofoam peanuts. Then she stretched the empty skins over their new, nondegradable bodies and stitched up the seams. Sometimes she gave them little black glass eyes, but often she used oversized, colored eyes like the kind you might find in a small doll. These she would stuff into their tiny polypropylene skulls and cut back the eyelids to allow for maximum exposure of the irises.

She spent hours designing tiny costumes. She made court jesters, pirates, racecar drivers, Jesus, a UPS deliveryman, and, at my insistence, Sally Jesse Raphael. Then she glued them to jelly-jar lids and placed the smartly dressed corpses at the mouths of all the little mouse holes around the tree house. Within weeks her problem was solved. The invading mice were appropriately creeped out by their mummified cousins in degrading costumes. Rather than risk suffering the same fate for a taste of quinoa or meatless beef-jerky, they scavenged for food elsewhere.

But Maple Jennifer had no desire to close her little taxidermy shop. Despite being a vegan, she had a natural affinity for killing and stuffing animals. It was yin and yang, her duality. Maple was unconflicted.

She took more classes and must have stuffed a hundred mice. I could see a definite progression in her work. The early specimens were lumpy and lopsided. Their coats were shoddily stitched and their outfits ill-fitting. By mouse number fifty, they looked as lovely and sprightly as any live mouse in a red satin bra and panties ever could.

My father never met Mapliffer or visited the tree house commune. Had he, I think he might have committed me to a mental institution. Besides the fact that I wanted to live like a Keebler elf, he would never have understood how I could pay rent for a place without a toilet. The fact that the toilet was only fifty yards down the path would only reinforce his fears that I'd lost my cotton-picking mind.

My parents were simply not from a socioeconomic group that understood choosing to live like an Irish immigrant fleeing the potato famine. They were proud and respectable people who worked hard for comfort and, more important, security. Initially, they found my behavior perplexing. Eventually, they realized that I was just like all the other unambitious kids at my mostly white prep school. I had no fear of the world. I had never worked hard on anything more important than a term paper. The world was a playground and I was ready to fall off every safety-engineered structure onto the recycled tennis shoe–padded ground. I wasn't conscious of white people. They were nothing more than a curious experiment in self-satisfaction. My privileged upbringing had instilled in me a sense of entitlement that didn't need reinforcing. That is really the American dream—not working hard and buying things, but reaching a place where there is no pressure to acknowledge that you already have everything.

The question was, how long could I keep everything when I didn't really deserve anything? And what did I have to do to be deserving? Would I be forced to contribute? It was fate and yet another whim that led me toward the answer to these questions.

I was either working as a disgruntled rug repairer or just back from a game show job in England when my sister said she was going to take the CBEST, a basic skills test required to become a teacher in California. At the time the state was so desperate for teachers that you could qualify for your own classroom, unsupervised, without even one minute of training. That was just the level of preparation I was looking for. We both signed up and three months later were employees of a local Unified School District. My sister was assigned a third grade class and I became an eighth grade English and U.S. history teacher at a middle school, just thirty miles away from the private academy where I'd gone to eighth grade, but worlds apart.

The school was blue. Every surface, without rhyme or reason, was painted a different shade of blue, except for my classroom, a portable at the far end of the main building that was painted in progressively degraded shades of thousand island dressing. The structure itself was made almost entirely of water-damaged particleboard wallpapered with faded construction paper. The only source of nonfluorescent light was through a small window in the door. Sometimes between classes I'd press my nose against that little rectangle of glass and stare at the dusty patch of dirt outside my door. The place made me want to kill myself.

My students were well-intentioned but had a fairly myopic view of the world. The girls would say things like "I'm going to have a baby when I'm sixteen and then go to junior college and marry a doctor." They'd be incredulous when I informed them that normal doctors don't cruise community colleges looking for stretched-out, low-aspiring girls with bastard children.

I spent a lot of time trying to expose them to reality, get them away from the television and the toxic microcosm that is middle school. I took one class hiking in the regional park. I explained that the paths weren't paved, that they needed sensible shoes, and not to dress in anything they wanted to wear again. Despite the cold, rainy day half the girls showed up in white platform sneakers, bell-bottoms, and bare-midriff shirts. Within minutes everybody's shoes were ruined or lost, having been sucked off their feet in the thick mud. I passed out garbage bags to wear as ponchos, but it wasn't until near hypothermia set in that the girls deigned to wear them. Then they pouted and sulked and cursed me.

Of the ten students in my group, six of them cried hysterically at some point during the afternoon. Some cried because they were scared of heights. "But we're on the ground. This is hardly even a hill." Others cried because of the wild turkeys, which were admittedly rather imposing birds, but also easily intimidated and skittish. One kid got crippling leg cramps and cried like he'd been shot. Others cried for their mamas, afraid we were lost like the Donner party and would soon resort to eating each other to survive. "But you can see the parking lot from here. We're only fifteen minutes from school."

After our hike, as we sat around eating pizza delivered from Domino's, the kids confided that they'd never been this far out in nature, with the wild animals. "Really?" I said. "I thought you were Lewis and Clark." They made other admissions during a game called Two Truths One Lie, ones that were surprising due to both intimacy and content. One boy said he saw his mother naked regularly. Another boy said he watched porn every morning, which explained why he was always late to my first-period class. And a girl said that her father used to be a pimp. "But don't tell anyone!"

"Sweetie," I said, "you cannot possibly think any of these fourteen-year-olds is going to keep that secret?"

When it was my turn to play I admitted that I'd hit my ex-boyfriend on the head with a frying pan. Of course, I followed it with a lecture on how violence is bad. I kept "unless he spent seventy dollars out of your wallet on a happy ending from a massage parlor" to myself.

Parents also needed some frank conversation regarding their children and I was happy to provide it, especially when required to stay after hours for parent-teacher conferences.

"Danny says you'll only let him submit questions in writing."

"That's right."

"Even during class? He's supposed to pass you a note with his question?"

"Yes, he sits in the front row specifically for that purpose."

"He says you said it's to keep him from asking, quote unquote, stupid questions."

"Yes," then a long stretch of silence while her eyebrows shot all over her forehead.

"But there is no such thing as a stupid question."

"Danny is full of stupid questions." More stunned silence. "Would you like some examples?"

She nodded.

"Asking what page we're on when the handout is only one page."

"I just don't think you should use the word *stupid*."

"What should I use?"

"How about *rhetorical*?"

"Rhetorical questions are asked to make a point. The only point Danny is making is that he isn't thinking. Writing the questions down forces Danny to think before he opens his mouth. You might want to try it . . . at home."

My class spent a lot of time goal setting, researching, and devising a life plan. We talked about the things they wanted, put price tags on them, figured out the requisite salaries and jobs that could provide the income necessary. Then we talked about personal strengths and weaknesses and made outlines so they could achieve their goals. It was an English-slash–*What Color Is Your Parachute?* class taught by the most unqualified teacher imaginable.

One day a smart-assed little punk raised his hand and said, "Ms. Norton, you obviously haven't dreamed your whole life of being an English teacher and driving that hoopty car. What do you want to be when you grow up?" Much like myself, my fourteen-year-old students didn't really grasp the fact that I was, in fact, already thirty years old.

Without hesitation I answered, "An astronaut."

"Then why aren't you an astronaut?"

The answer was complicated. Everything I'd just told them,

about how life is not complicated and people just try to make it that way when they don't want to do what they need to do, was bullshit. They could take their little binder pages filled with inspirational notes about goals and overcoming obstacles, about being persistent and not making excuses or illegitimate children, and wipe their pimpled little behinds with them. I started to mutter something about being bad at math, but it was just lame. So I said, "I happen to really love that car."

But the little masturbator was absolutely right, so after school that day, after sending more military boarding school applications to his house, I started doing some research and found a local state school where I could do some post-bac science work and finally fulfill my dream of becoming the world's most unlikely astronaut.

The next day I sat down with my class and wrote a plan for myself that I posted over the board. If I was going to use class time for my own self-improvement I might as well put it under the guise of helping the students. The first thing I needed to do was review trigonometry in preparation for calculus. I soon learned that I needed to review algebra in preparation for trig. Then I realized that I needed to review my multiplication tables in preparation for algebra. (I should have known as a third grader that cheating with a pocket calculator behind my mother's back as she simultaneously quizzed me and prepared dinner would come back to haunt me. Now, here I was, twenty-something years later with little flash cards that read six times seven is forty-two.)

By the time I got to my algebra review I knew I needed help. I recruited some of the more advanced eighth graders to tutor me. They found it immensely amusing that their teacher couldn't factor a square, remember exponent rules, or add fractions. But I persevered, and within weeks was as competent as any thirteen-year-old.

I was finally ready to begin my trig class at the university. Surprisingly, Euclidian trigonometry had changed significantly since I took it in eleventh grade. What was all this sine, cosine, and tangent nonsense? What was a matrix and how could I ever figure out an equation with five variables? It seemed to me that if you needed to answer a question with five variables, you should gather a bit more information.

Unfortunately, the teacher was something between totally useless and worthy of contempt. He assigned four hours of homework a night, yet he couldn't explain anything. He never returned our corrections and quizzed us on uncovered topics. On our final exam, for which only eight of the original forty students showed up, the first question was unsolvable by design. We all wasted twenty minutes on an unplottable graph. When somebody asked if he had tried to solve it, he smirked and said, "Not all questions have answers," to which the habitually silent, chubby guy in the last row responded: "You prick."

It wasn't until this class that I realized my self-confidence might be overconfidence. This was a California state school. Anybody with a high school diploma who applied was accepted. I had graduated on the dean's list from Columbia (not exactly summa cum laude, but respectable). This little state school should have been easy. What I was learning was that what separates the Ivy League student body from the state school student body is economics, not intelligence. I found myself surrounded by poor and lower-middle-class kids desperate to pull themselves up by their bootstraps and willing to study eight hours a day to do it. My cocktail party banter proved useless in my chemistry classes. Knowing the differences between Kant and Kublia Khan did not help calculate torque and friction. I woke up one morning and decided that I needed to justify my superiority complex.

And I definitely had a superiority complex, stemming from one defining moment that made me think I was better than everybody else. Rockridge Elementary, kindergarten, 1975. My family had moved from South San Francisco to Oakland and I started at a new school halfway through the year. Not only could I already read, had been able to for years, and ride a two-wheel bike, but I could draw horses and realistic hands even in ink.

The classroom had two pet rats that the kids built mazes for and sometimes took home on weekends. They had stupid names like Cheesy and Fuzzy that the whole class had chosen democratically before my arrival. I decided the names should be changed to Panther and Plague, after the Black Panthers, also from Oakland, and the black death, transmitted by fleas on rats, two facts my father had recently shared with me. This white teacher in a fairly multicultural school in the early '70s was understandably reluctant to bring race politics into the kindergarten classroom, and felt that the bubonic plague was something five-year-olds could learn about later. She denied my renaming request, saying that the names they had were more appropriate.

Mutiny was the only choice so I began a campaign to

change the names ourselves, without Mrs. No Imagination's permission. Cheesy and Fuzzy were baby names and the teacher wanted to treat us like babies. If we wanted to be widespread death-obsessed, black power militant big kids, the names had to go. Within hours the whole kindergarten class was addressing the rodents as I wished. Mrs. Kaye continued calling them by their old names until she sounded pathetic. It only took a day or two, and then even the nameplates on their cages were replaced. No trace of Fuzzy or Cheesy remained. I remember walking home with my neighbor Isa and marveling at how easy it was to manipulate those dummies. I knew then how malleable the world was and how powerful I could be. I didn't even need to use my power, but I had it.

That power I felt back then, and had grown so comfortable with over the years, now felt more like delusion. I sat in every lecture, read every page, went to every lab, and was far from mastering any subject, or even appearing to. Other students were outperforming me, and I was trying as hard as I could. True failure, not the kind where you just give up, but the kind where you try and try and never succeed, was a real possibility here. Maybe my doing a half-assed job wasn't just an affectation. Maybe it was all I could do. Luckily, the people with means, the people who surrounded me, always filled in that last little bit, the bit that made me quirky and charming. Without them, and their resources, I was just another mediocre, talentless black girl without a savings account.

If my luck ran out I wouldn't be playing with granola girl and living in a tree house; I'd be living permanently in the projects. That might be a great adventure for me, getting to know all those colorful ghetto characters and answering the big questions, like why does Ray Ray ride his bike all day? How come June Bug always wears her slippers outside, and why isn't there a grocery store within three miles, but there are eighteen liquor stores? But if I raised my kids there, they'd just be ghetto kids. They'd see hookers in the middle of the day. They would be afraid of dogs. They'd spend thirty thousand dollars on a car before they made a down payment on a house. This was the realization I had at Cal State Hayward, right before I met Thibault, gathered up my junk, had a baby, decided to stop being so damned capricious and make something of myself.

This was the realization I had again when my father told me my cancer was the worst thing that ever happened to him. He'd put in so much hard work, sacrificed so much, and I was going to expire before I'd come into my own. My father loves me for the dilettante I am, but his pride rides on my potential, and I was going to die long before realizing it.

chapter seventeen

The survival statistics on inflammatory breast cancer, 40 percent after five years, and worse after metastasis, led me to believe that the standard treatment was hardly the wonder cure patients prayed for. Granted, it was considerably more successful than the previous regimen that prescribed surgery before chemotherapy. Those results were so poor that if you actually lived five years they concluded that you had been misdiagnosed. These improved odds, though, were only slightly better than flipping a coin.

After three months of chemo, with less than stellar results, I became convinced that nobody had any idea what they were doing. Sure my doctors were well trained and my tumor was certainly smaller, but it was still there. I had pain in my arm, meaning my lymph nodes were probably still affected. And the skin on my breast remained thick and dimply. We weren't doing enough.

I needed information. Why hadn't a single physician recommended that I alter my diet? I'd read enough books to know that your immune system is greatly influenced by what you eat. I also knew that cancer is a malfunction of your immune system. Why wasn't this correlation being addressed? Cancer cells love refined sugar. Why were my chemo nurses offering me cup after cup of sweetened juice? And sticky buns? And jelly beans full of carcinogenic red dye? Why did I have to ask three times for a referral to the nutritionist? When I did see her, why did she just stare at me blankly and, like an android, repeat again and again that I was not to lose weight during chemotherapy?

My father the doctor tried to calm me by defending doctors. He said that they were extremely knowledgeable, highly trained professionals. I should trust them, but they were also mere mortals, not gods. I already knew this, having grown up surrounded by doctors, friends of my parents, and friends of my own. These people couldn't parallel park or set the clock on the VCR. My father could fashion a woman out of a man, but couldn't make rice. My friend Anne operated on babies in utero, but actually married a guy who stole her checkbook, twice, before the wedding. Why couldn't my father have been a stockbroker and my friends professional skateboarders so I could still have the appropriate awe to feel really confident?

We like to pretend that our physicians leave the office, attend a seminar, eat a healthy dinner hosted by a drug manufacturer, and then relax at home with some medical journals. They don't. Usually they're just glad to be around people who aren't dying or spewing germs or needing abscesses drained. They listen to Howard Stern, yell at their children, and don't always use paper liners in public toilets. They are flawed people, subject to bad judgment and folly just like the rest of us.

My father stopped short of saying that unlike the rest of us, whose work screwup might mean needing another Xerox toner cartridge, doctor screwups mean maiming, paralysis, and the death of your daughter. Doctoring is just their job; some of them suck at it, at least once in a while. Finally he was on the other side of the desk and saw just how terrifying trusting a stranger with your life really is. He saw just how desperately I needed total confidence in these people, even when that confidence was dependent on their admitting they didn't know what they were doing or why one thing worked and another didn't. I didn't expect miracles, just the truth, and no mistakes.

The instant I convinced my father that my points were valid was the instant the clinical professor in him kicked in. The next appointment we had, he drilled Dr. Ree as if she were one of his residents. He had a stack of studies and a list of questions and launched into her.

"The immunoperoxidase panel . . . sentinel node biopsy . . . residual infiltration . . ." She answered each of his questions concisely in a controlled voice.

"What about a nonsurgical approach? Have you considered that?" His tone grew more combative.

Dr. Ree's voice stayed controlled, but her clenched fists betrayed her defensiveness. "Some reports suggest higher locoregional failure rates—"

"Locoregional!? And what effect does that have on overall survival? I don't give a damn about local control! Overall survival!"

Nothing good would come of this conversation. My father was about to rupture something and we were well on our way to alienating the best breast surgeon in the area.

"It is simply not acceptable!" My father was not using his indoor voice.

"Dr. Norton!" He'd found her limit, but before she could finish her rebuttal Daddy broke down sobbing.

"It is simply not acceptable that Meredith is one of the sixty percent, the ones that don't make it."

Dr. Ree covered my father's big brown surgeon's hand with her own little peach-colored one, a gesture far more effective than anything she could have said.

We would trust this doctor with my life, not because she was qualified and handled my father, but because we had to trust someone. I couldn't do this particular job for myself. I'd chosen to herd pygmy goats in Minorca while she went to medical school. She did the training, passed the exams, got the degrees, and had the authority to pump me full of toxins and chop off my breasts. I had no choice but to lie still and trust she wasn't too distracted by her house's termite problem to confuse me with the lobotomy patient at 9:30. All doctors are people, even though we wish they were something better.

The best I could do was educate myself before I ended up on one of those medical mistake talk shows. People had been sending me articles and journals and I'd just piled them all into an unread heap. It was time to crack a few books and figure out just what this locally advanced breast cancer was.

It took half an hour of reading to realize my entire treatment was based on one assumption: my diagnosis. How did I know that I really had cancer? They could have said lupus or shingles or anything. I needed to meet with the pathologist and see my biopsy slides for myself.

The pathology department matched the overall dreariness of the rest of the hospital, but lacked the failed attempts at charm found in the other offices. It was clearly not intended to be viewed or even found by the patients. Only those willing to explore the darkest, hidden basement corridors, passing through doors marked "Hazardous Waste" and "Radioactive" could ever find it. It was not nice. There was no waiting room, no anxiety-reducing fish tank. I was ushered into the conference room by a clearly befuddled assistant who kept asking me what department I was from and addressing me as doctor. On the table lay a smattering of highly graphic autopsy photos and opened textbooks with diagrams of unrecognizable body parts and captions in Latin. I was thrilled. By the time the pathologist interrupted me, I was fully engrossed in penile malformations and accompanying glandular dysfunction—a subject with which I was not thoroughly unfamiliar, having had an absentminded urologist for a father. As a child, the textbooks and instructional videos that littered the house were better than pornography and I perused them greedily. It did not take long to become quite knowledgeable on the subjects of castration, penectomy, metoidioplasty (sex change), as well as the logistics of the vasectomy and benefits of prostate milking. In sixth grade I probably knew more about vesicoureteral reflux than most medical school students.

The pathologist who appeared was a sultry, albeit bookish woman. She showed me my biopsy slides, and explained ductal carcinoma and staging. It was absolutely fascinating and after she stopped stuttering, calling the specimen "y-y-you" and just went with "the patient," I started to really enjoy myself. I even started to feel proud.

My cancer cells were extraordinary. They were exceptionally strong and well formed. The nuclei were enormous and the borders grossly misshapen. In fact, it was the erratic borders that were evidence of why this cancer was so lethal and aggressive. The more harmless a cancer, the more organized it is. The more organized it is, the easier it is to decode and destroy. My special cancer was so chaotic and berserk that it couldn't even organize itself enough to form a tumor. It just spread arbitrarily in any direction. Like a crowd of looters, it was difficult to contain and control, especially since the doctors had no real understanding of the source of the riot. My cancer, like an old dog, resembled its owner. It was my bloodthirsty little doppelgänger.

The pathologist's argument was convincing and I agreed that I did indeed have cancer. That was one thing less to doubt. Next, I needed to figure out why 60 percent of patients were dying from this form of it and how not to join them. I needed to find the loophole, my true talent.

I dove into my stack of articles with all the zeal someone in her thirteenth week of chemotherapy could muster. I knew that being in control of my treatment was the only way to survive. My whole life I knew that if you want something done right, you have to do it yourself. I took this to heart when it came to cake decorating, pedicures, and orgasms, but suddenly, when my life depended on it, I couldn't maintain the enthusiasm I needed.

I tried many times to research, but either grew bored by the simplistic explanations to my questions or got hopelessly distracted by minutiae. Finding comprehensive answers that weren't insulting to my intelligence was difficult. One site actually said, "Adriamycin kills quickly dividing (reproducing) tumor cells (bad cells) while allowing healthy (good) cells to survive." And worse than being condescending, this information was inaccurate. Adriamycin kills any dividing cell, healthy or not. Hence, my bald head.

Even on the rare occasion that I did find a good site, I couldn't focus my attention on it. I'd be reading a study that took place in Helsinki and end up spending two hours googling the Finnish girl I'd met years ago on a train in Yugoslavia. Once I spent four hours trying to find pictures of Pygmy people to see just how tiny they really were. I found plenty of pictures, but the people were never juxtaposed to anything scalable. I saw Pygmies standing next to trees, but who knew how big the trees were? At the end of the day I was thoroughly frustrated and no closer to understanding either my disease or tiny Africans.

I couldn't even blame my attention deficit on chemo brain. I'd always been this way, it just never mattered before. As a teacher I was once handing out prep papers for a state-mandated standardized test. As I passed one to this little Filipino kid named Juan, I noticed the outrageously huge, pronounced, ripe field of blackheads that filled every pore within a two-inch radius of his nostrils. It was more like an oval, with the nostrils as the double foci. They were jet black, greasy lubed, and so ready to squeeze that I forgot completely about the exam. The kids had to remind me several times that time had run out, the twenty minutes for the analytical skills section had passed, because I was too busy staring at Juan's acne and daydreaming about all the implausible scenarios that allowed me to free the hardened, oxidized pus from the poor boy's nose.

But this time I wasn't being distracted from some irrelevant test that determined our school's funding for the next year, I was being distracted from saving my own life. And while my digressions often led to amusing trivia, they rarely yielded really useful information. I had the serious charge to cure myself and it required my buckling down and learning. There were no loopholes here. These were brass tacks.

It was too late to do anything about chemo, being almost done, so I decided to focus on the next stage of treatment: surgery. When surgery was the only form of treatment, a monotherapy, everyone died. Even when they followed it with chemotherapy, everyone died. And with radiation, everyone died. But they discovered that if they started with chemo, then did surgery and radiation, more people lived, like . . . somebody. I deduced that this meant the problem was surgery. Surgery must activate something that caused the disease to metastasize. Only with total systemic control in the beginning could one actually survive the surgery and live for more than a year or two.

I went on the Internet and sought information to support what I wanted to hear, namely that I did not need a mastectomy. As with virtually every subject, medical, political, or sexual, one can find a league of supporters on the Internet. For every breed of deviant freak there is an international club that meets bimonthly in cyberspace, which is actually the problem with the Internet. Any aberrant whim is instantly gratified, or at least acknowledged and further encouraged. There is no good reason to lie naked with your cat, and certainly no reason to make it a community practice, but nudist cat fanciers have a Web site that gets hundreds of hits weekly.

I could certainly find, and did, physicians successfully treating IBC without surgery. I sent copies of their published studies to my doctors. We had meeting after phone call after memo and I just could not convince them that surgery was unnecessary. They pointed out that my grasp of statistics was superficial at best, if they were willing to admit I had any grasp of statistics at all. There is a whole field of medical statistics that people study for years in order to devise treatment protocols. I was simply being naive to disregard them and put so much faith in myself.

The last time I had been called "naive" was January 2, 2000. The period of naïveté actually began four days earlier in Seville, Spain, where my friend Jenny and I got into a car crash. It was entirely my fault as I was badmouthing Asian drivers when I miscalculated a turn and skidded into oncoming traffic. We hit a Fiat Panda head-on, and in addition to breaking a trunk load of hand-painted ceramics we'd just picked up in Lisbon, I slammed my chin on the steering wheel and chipped all my teeth, top and bottom. Jenny had pretty serious whiplash and both cars were totaled, but the rental company did not hesitate to offer us an immediate replacement when we limped into their office completely traumatized. We declined and continued by train, and then ferry to Morocco, where we planned to spend the Y2K New Year's Eve.

I remember very little of the trip across the Strait of Gibraltar because my chipped teeth were driving me crazy. Not only were they hypersensitive to heat, cold, and texture, but they were sharp like broken glass. I couldn't resist constantly touching them and, consequently, had a swollen, bloody, shredded tongue that was useless regarding anything practical, like eating.

After checking into a hotel in Fez I asked the concierge if he could recommend a dentist. His response was: "Absolutely not." I explained my issue, showed him my tongue, at which sight he cringed. I asked him again. "Absolutely not."

"I just need to get them filed. They're sharp."

"Look at the others' teeth." He had a point there. I hadn't seen a full mouth of healthy teeth in an adult since I'd stepped off the boat at Tangier. Mostly people had a combination of yellow, brown, and black stumps juxtaposed with gaping holes. "You wait until you get back to Spain."

"I can't wait. Look at my tongue. It is unbearable. Please, help me find a dentist."

"You are naive," he said. "A woman like you is no match for a dentist."

Challenged, Jenny and I trawled the souk, the walled maze of tiny streets and alleys that made up the ancient city, despite the concierge's warning against it. "Two foreign women alone will never find their way." What was this guy's issue with women? After a couple of hours we found a dentist's office, or assumed so by the curio cabinet of secondhand dentures for sale displayed in the alley outside.

We entered the office, which was no more than a single room with a very used-looking dentist chair and a reading light suspended from the ceiling. Next to the chair was a rusty metal table with some huge, and very primitive-looking tools laid out on top of it. The dentist stood, mouth agape, in the corner. He appeared to either have all of his teeth or a very

123

convincing set of false ones, so Jenny and I attempted, in four languages, to explain my predicament. Knowing the word for *file* in French, German, Spanish, or Arabic would have been helpful, but pantomime sufficed in its absence.

The dentist assured me that he understood and helped me into the chair. I opened my mouth and he probed around, mumbling all the while. Then he reached for a blue plastic bottle and sprayed the most potent, bleach-based antiseptic into my mouth. I howled as it burned into the dozens of tiny lacerations on my tongue. Then he reached for the pliers and I sat bolt upright. He pushed me back down. Jenny ran to my side. He pushed her back. "Whoa, dude, just file them. File them. No, no, no, no pliers."

He held me down with one arm and the weight of his body and with the other hand tried to push the pliers past my clenched teeth. Jenny was screaming at him and pushing and finally waved her U.S. passport just inches from his face. That stunned him long enough that I broke free and jumped to my feet panting. He seemed genuinely surprised. "No pull my teeth, man. File them, make smooth, smooth." Jenny was pulling me toward the door, but I saw a rasp on his table and knew if I could only show him he could help me. I took the rasp, poured some of the bleach on it, and filed the sharpest points as he looked on in amazement. I honestly think he had no idea there was any dental treatment besides extraction. I had indeed been naive. One woman was no match for a dentist. It took two of us and the full intimidation factor of the U.S. government.

If the concierge was right then, maybe the doctors were

right now. This was no time to be naive with the stakes so high. I needed a fourth opinion. I found a doctor in San Francisco who was familiar with the studies I'd read. She examined them and talked with me for over an hour before concluding that I shouldn't stray from my doctors' suggestions. She was condescending, saying that I really shouldn't draw conclusions because as a layperson there was no way I could understand the scientific language of medical journals. There was so much information that any conclusions I reached could only be done so from the most superficial data.

How stupid did she think I was? Of course medical jargon is complicated and confusing. That is why I had a medical dictionary. Plus, I was hardly going to pretend I understood something I didn't when my own life depended on it. "How could you," she said, "possibly understand the complicated mechanics of cell biology?"

"Look," I said lying, "I am getting a PhD in aerospace engineering! I can make a helicopter out of your desk."

"Too bad that won't cure your cancer."

"Touché."

Dealing with people in such situations can never be easy, but Dr. Ree seemed to have unlimited patience. I have no doubt she wanted to block my e-mail and refuse my calls, but she never did. She scheduled appointment after appointment with my father and me. She listened to all my rantings and justifications for why I wouldn't follow the prescribed course of treatment. Not once did she scream, "You moron with your Internet medical degree! Stop questioning me!" She just nodded her head when I canceled my surgery and thought to herself, "You poor, stupid dolt." Then she quietly rescheduled it when I called her back.

Other doctors weren't so amenable. When I changed my mind regarding surgery the second time, Dr. Yuen stamped her foot in frustration and asked, "We already discussed this! What is wrong with you?" Oh, I don't know. Maybe I'm terrified of dying and leaving my one-year-old with no memory of his mother. When I told her the third time that I was refusing surgery and just using radiation for local control, she stifled a scream and then I think pounded her head against the wall. My new oncologist actually called me up and said, "Do you want to die?! Do you want to die?!" when I considered refusing further treatment entirely.

Eventually, all the doctors got together, intervention style, with Dr. Ree as spokeswoman, and explained that they absolutely did not believe my self-prescribed course of nontreatment was prudent, but would support my decision. It was a patient's right to refuse treatment. Then they looked at me as though it was for the last time, eyes drooped with disappointment, truly sad that I was so stupid and going to die soon, and that they'd missed the coffee and pastry cart for this pointless meeting.

"Whatever." I was immune to their reverse psychology. "Could somebody please forward my chart?"

Unfortunately, there was no place to forward my chart to. After talking to the doctor leading the only reputable study of treatment without surgery, I learned that he wouldn't enroll me. I hadn't responded well enough to chemotherapy. After four months, there was still too much disease obviously present to think it could be eradicated with radiation alone. If he were in my shoes, he said, he'd get rid of that breast as soon as possible.

I felt like my friend who married a terror. As soon as she accepted his proposal and set a wedding date his grandmother called, insisting that she sign a prenuptial agreement. Her fiancé supported her and the two of them fought off the matriarch's pressure. My friend was so distracted by this insult and the ensuing battle that she forgot to remember what a demented freak her future husband was and why it had taken her two weeks to accept the stunningly gorgeous, two-carat canary diamond engagement ring. At the reception the grandmother took her aside and admitted that this had never been about the contract; she just wanted to keep the new bride's mind off the real issue: her grandson's mental illness.

Distraction or not, I had raised a few legitimate questions, ones that would influence my later treatments. But overall this whole thing had served to make me feel less passive. One of the first things I realized about this process is that I was just along for the ride. Cancer isn't like a cyst that you can massage away. I couldn't set aside forty minutes a day to treat myself. Some people try to do just that. They sit down and visualize their bodies killing cancer cells. They use meditation to put them in control of this microscopic battle.

For me, those techniques did not work. I tried to envision soldier cells slaying cancer cells, one by one. My mind would instead wander to action films like *Braveheart* and *Troy* where the soldiers had on little skirts and no underwear. Did the real William Wallace paint his face blue? What kind of paint did he use? Whatever was available in the thirteenth century was either toxic or permanent. And that would make me think about the Bayeux Tapestry. The audiotape at the museum described every stupid little battle but neglected to address the naked guys wrestling pigs and sodomizing each other in the lower frieze. And that would make me think about the things people never explain, because they just don't know, which is why 60 percent of IBC patients are still dying. Then I'd be all worked up and back to attacking the doctors.

I was going to have to slink back, all lame and pathetic, to Dr. Ree and ask yet again to be put on her surgery schedule. Could I just live long enough to learn how to avoid these situations? With as much disease as I had present, probably not.

My return to Dr. Ree's care was more like the belly flop that punctuates a flailing dive, but she put on her flashiest Chris smile—she's the sexiest of Charlie's Angels—and penciled me in for a mastectomy. She appeared to be pleased, but at this point I think all the doctors were actually hoping I would die just to get out of their hair, or at least continue my treatment elsewhere so they could spend their hours dealing with patients who showed proper respect.

I sent cards in beautiful, un-return-addressed envelopes so the doctors would have to read my apology before realizing it was from the crazy girl and her father. It seemed to work, and by my next visit all seemed forgiven. I was free again to lounge around guiltlessly and focus on myself.

chapter eighteen

Nonappointment days were spent in our one-room house. I was either in bed sleeping, or watching from bed as Thibault played with Lucas, or peering from bed to the kitchen to oversee Thibault's cooking, or eating in bed. I sometimes got out of bed to avoid bedsores and walk really lazily down the driveway to the mailbox, or the *magische Perückemaschine* (German for "magic wig machine"), as we grew to call it.

I found at least two wigs in the mailbox every week; my cancer seemed like just the excuse everybody in the world needed to send me recycled hair. There were also lots of hats: sunhats, caps, bonnets, and even a couple of those turbans rich widows from Palm Springs wear to see their lawyers. I got frozen food, ostrich feathers, tulip bulbs, and lots of books. There were books on gardening, will writing, diet, and Lance Armstrong. There were lots of books by Lance Armstrong (written with a ghostwriter, or *nègre,* as the French call them. Typical to call the person who does all the labor, like building America, but gets none of the credit, a black), although they were mostly copies of one book, *Every Second Counts.*

Spending time experiencing someone else's life when your own appears about to run out seemed like a poor choice, so, besides the required medical journals and nutrition books, I rarely read at all. It was a day or two before my final chemo appointment and Thibault had taken Lucas out when I finally picked up one of Lance's books.

Actually, I stared at the cover picture for quite a while. Lance is there, holding his son, both smiling. They are in the foreground, but shadowed and dark. It's a classic example of why you use a flash in the sunlight. Behind the Armstrongs is a crowd, well lit but blurry. Three guys look directly into the camera. One, in particular, a sort of fat-faced French guy with a big nose and small mouth, is almost craning to get into the picture. I identified more with this guy and the associated fame of being a head filling in the background of this famous photo than with Lance Armstrong, the cancer icon and family man.

For a while there was a picture of me on the Columbia College home page for student life. I was sitting on the library steps looking perfectly collegiate. The funniest thing is I'd only done that once in my whole four years at Columbia. I was supposed to meet this guy I was all gaga over. Henry Pincus was into acting, lived off-campus, and looked like Tom Cruise, all intense. He was exactly the kind of boy I can't stand in a man. I'd been working on the seduction for months, literally since the first day of classes in September. It was now mid-April. Finally, he was taking me to lunch. He showed up thirty minutes late. I waited, reading some dreadful textbook, posing with my shoes off, in an effort not to look frantic. I wanted to throw myself down the granite steps and die.

When he did make his appearance, all full of lame apologies, I told him I'd have to take a rain check. Never being one of those transparently hurt girls, either hypervulnerable or stinking of bravado, I was all smiles and apologies myself. I had simply forgotten a meeting with a professor or some such nonsense. We chatted for ten minutes, me staring at my watch the whole time; then I raced off to take the long route to my dorm room and practice my married signature: Mrs. Henry Pincus. Later we did start seeing each other and I drove him crazy. By the end he couldn't stand the sight of me and actually called me tiresome.

That one guy, just to the left of Lance Armstrong's head, the one looking straight into the camera, was he really into cycling or was he looking for that wench who had stood him up? It was Paris, maybe he'd just stepped in *merde,* and that's why he had such a somber expression. Things are rarely as they seem.

As soon as I started reading the book, I had problems with it. For starters, Lance Armstrong and I are the same age, yet he seems like an adult, and I don't. Nobody would describe him as a kid. He isn't asking his parents to pay his health insurance. He doesn't still debate what he's going to be when he grows up. I doubt that he looks at his own kids and wonders when their real parents are going to pick them up. And he certainly can't still be stealing toothpaste and toilet paper from his mom's house. He has probably never short-sheeted his in-laws' bed.

Maybe it is because I had such a fabulous childhood—long summer vacations and big slumber parties, no worries, no responsibilities—that I couldn't leave childhood behind. My family was as nuclear as they come. My mother did everything she was supposed to do. She sat down with us and checked our homework. She made three perfectly balanced meals every day, which we all ate together. She corrected our grammar. My father came home from work at precisely six o'clock with briefcase in hand. Nobody got molested or teen pregnant. We all got cars when we turned sixteen. There was no drama outside of the acceptable sibling rivalry. My parents kept their disagreements behind closed and soundproof doors. Our family lived the ideal that there is just a certain way things are done. We all played our respective parts and lived comfortably in our Cosby cocoon. Nothing bad ever happened to us.

When I was twelve my sister, Angela, was sixteen and desperate to get a job. I looked at her like she had a KFC biscuit for a brain. Why on Earth would she want to grow up so fast? She had a lifetime of conference rooms and expense reports and panty hose ahead of her. Why would she want to bring that drudgery into her life while she could still be making cookies in her Easy-Bake Oven and watching *Pippi Longstocking* with her friends?

Not that I didn't work. I worked my skinny little ass off—having two jobs at once for years here and there. I just would have preferred not to. And I never made any progress toward a career. My job limit was always three years. I worked at working in production for three years, taught for three years, ran my pillow company for three years. I never kept with any job long enough to become accomplished. Whatever promise I showed early on, I never persevered long enough to be successful. Hence, my second problem with Lance Armstrong: Lance Armstrong is adept at everything he does, at least publicly. Perhaps he is a failed potter in the privacy of his own basement. He has been successful in business, triathlons, bicycle racing, and celebrity. In his book he tells the reader again and again that he works harder than everybody else and that is why his results are superior. Even during chemo he rode his bike five hours a day. Now, chemo was not hard on me. Compared to most patients, I had it easy. That said, if I could walk through Target and then stay up past eight o'clock, I felt like a rock star.

One evening I went dancing at the veterans' center, a senior citizens' club that has weekly ballroom dancing for octogenarians and their parents. I thought that I could at least hang out with these old guys for a few hours. They tucked me in and turned out the lights. One veteran of the War of 1812 complained that his having to drag me around the floor like a wet sack of sand was going to aggravate his phlebitis. He kept clicking his dentures at me like some ornery squirrel. It was exhausting. He might have shuffled in on a walker, but once they got that gramophone spinning he seriously perked up.

Lance Armstrong has excessive drive and talent. His motivation and discipline grow like crab grass and dandelions. I just don't have it like that. Every day of my chemo that I ate a Krispy Kreme doughnut or took a nap instead of doing yoga I cursed Lance Armstrong and his toned abs, tiny butt, and three kinds of cancer. "F you, Lance Armstrong," I muttered as I sucked down my Dr Pepper. "You can park your bike right here and kiss my ass."

Give me some fat slob on welfare who never graduated from junior high and can't ride around the block without choking on his cigarette, and yet manages to pull himself together, go macrobiotic, and beat cancer, and I will show you one inspired Meredith Norton.

chapter nineteen

The initial report that I needed a bilateral or double mastectomy was exaggerated. There was no evidence that I would develop any disease in the other breast. So, after the initial freak-out Dr. Ree and my father decided that a unilateral mastectomy would suffice. It made surprisingly little difference to me. What exactly was I meant to do with one goddamned breasticle? Stand sideways all the time and wear asymmetrical blouses?

I had lived my whole life as a flat-chested girl, spent summer after disappointing summer waiting for my breasts to sprout like all the other girls' had. Finally, during my thirty-third winter, as my son grew in my belly, conical, rock-hard breasts burst forth from my chest. To my own surprise, and the rest of my family's revulsion, I was one of those nursing women who whipped out her jugs any- and everywhere. Being that, even fully engorged with milk, I was only a C-cup, my breasts didn't really have that pendulous swing that draws serious attention. People would be startled to realize that while adoring my cherubic little son, they were inadvertently staring at my chocolaty nipple.

My male in-laws took a while to adjust. Even though French streets are wallpapered with images of naked bodies, full-on sexual intercourse with penetration is broadcast on television at all hours, and the beaches are littered with topless women and men in suspiciously lumpy Speedos, the practice of a woman exposing her breast to nourish her child is taboo. How dare I use my breasts as anything but sexual objects or a tool to sell toothpaste?

Once, when nursing Lucas at a café, a woman approached me. It was ten in the morning, the only hour I could enter a café without suffocating from the cigarette smoke. I had Lucas on my lap with my blouse discreetly unbuttoned from the bottom. Apparently, this was not discreet enough as this woman stood by my table—nasty cigarette hanging from her chapped gray lips smeared with greasy oxblood lipstick—and started to berate me. Foul-smelling smoke poured from her mouth and nostrils onto my baby and me. "How dare you," she said in her slurry Parisian French, "subject the public to your primitive rituals! There is no dignity left in France! In the world!"

I called her a dirty pervert, an insult at which she gasped, spun on her heels, and complained about to the waiter. He just laughed, looked at me, and explained to her that things were different in Africa.

During my mastectomy surgery the hospital lobby was packed with Meredith supporters and supporters of supporters. Pretty much everybody except Thibault and my father were sitting there. My father had convinced Thibault that after forty-odd years of practice, the only logical time to help him move out of his office was during the three hours his wife got her breast amputated. I like to pretend this was my father's way of helping Thibault cope by presenting a distraction. Unfortunately, I think he really wanted help and saw a window when he knew his son-in-law technically wasn't busy. Since

Thibault had agreed to help, and was incapable of saying "Piss off," he was forced to pack and unpack boxes filled with papers my father could shred at his leisure during his retirement instead of waiting at the hospital for his young wife, the mother of his toddler son, to have her deadly tumor removed.

According to Rebecca, when Thibault finally broke away and came to the hospital, he was such a wreck he could barely talk. They brought him immediately to see me in recovery and even gray/beige, the black version of pale, bundled head to toe in heated blankets, and sedated, I managed to boss him around even more, insisting that he give each of the doctors and nurses one of the nippled boob cupcakes I'd made the night before.

The mastectomy went so smoothly I didn't suffer even one minute of pain, which was a shame because I'd been looking forward to needing to relieve the pain with a nice narcotic. During labor I was given morphine and in one instant completely understood why people become drug addicts. The pain was still there, but I just didn't care because I was busy being warm and happy. Filthy crack houses, cockroaches, and societal scorn—all the bugaboos of being a junkie—seemed like a fair trade for the joyous rapture I felt when the nurse plunged the opiate into my IV drip.

It had been over a year since I experienced that level of pleasure and I was jonesing to feel so blank and cozy again. Only this time, unfortunately, there was no pain. I was sore, of course, but this was nothing like the twenty hours of contractions and the C-section I'd suffered through with Lucas. Eight hundred milligrams of Tylenol could have set me right.

Nevertheless, I lobbied for the real drugs. The nurse administered it and I almost cried from disappointment.

Not only was I not enveloped in the warm embrace of a drug-induced high, the disappointment was dampening the natural high I was already experiencing from having my husband and ex-fiancé and ex-boyfriend all visiting at the same time. There I sat on a mechanical, Posturepedic dais, bald and one-tittied, while the two exes rushed to fluff my pillows and Thibault studied my appearance, wondering if he had in fact won or lost. I should have been luxuriating in it, but instead I sat, frantically pumping the dosage button and worrying that my drainage bag would fall out of my gown and expose the bulb full of serum and lymph.

I stayed in the hospital for three days even though they said I could leave the day of the surgery. This was the first chance I'd had to be by myself since the diagnosis, and to sleep alone, no husband stealing the covers, no baby kicking me in the neck, since getting married. I felt like I was really on a vacation. I wasn't even encouraged to go out and play golf or swing on a trapeze. I could just stay in the room, read, watch television, and sleep. My nurses brought me food and changed my dressings and linens. My bed sat me up and laid me down. I had a nice, private room with a lovely view of the city. I didn't even have to be pleasant and chat up some roommate. It was blissful.

When I explained to the nurses that I didn't ever want to leave they looked at me like my labor-and-delivery nurse had when it was time to remove my catheter. I'd had it in for three days after my Cesarean and had grown to love it. It seems odd to adore a tube hanging from your crotch, attached to a plastic bag filled with warm urine, but I did. I'd spent the previous nine months running to the toilet every twenty minutes, day and night. The last two months I ran to the toilet and still peed on myself when I stood up afterward. It drove me crazy. Urinating effortlessly and at my leisure into a bag was downright luxurious. I didn't even have to empty the reservoir. It was hidden under my sheets and I completely forgot about it until the nurses came to whisk it away.

Dr. Ree had told me that my surgery would be the easiest part of my treatment. I thought it would be terribly painful and traumatic. I also had this crazy fear that I'd develop lymphedema. Lymphedema is caused when lymph nodes are removed or compromised and a limb is no longer able to regulate properly the flow of lymph, the waterlike fluid in which red blood cells are suspended. The swelling can be extreme, causing the arm or leg to bloat like a Ballpark frank. It is also painful, unsightly, and permanent.

I imagined myself with this huge right arm, all engorged like a Macy's Thanksgiving Day Parade penis balloon. I even bought a flesh-toned pressure sleeve designed to prevent the accumulation of fluid. When I put it on I couldn't bend my stupid arm and it cut off the circulation. I felt wholly unarticulated, like some cheap plastic doll. And not being able to bend my right elbow inexplicably caused me to stop bending my left elbow, both my knees, and my neck. I sort of swiveled at the waist like a Japanese robot from a *Godzilla* flick. I was even convinced that that damned sleeve was causing me to lose my peripheral vision. It was totally debilitating so I rarely wore the contraption.

I considered seeing a therapist about my extreme fear of lymphedema and complete unwillingness to prevent it, but was still put off by that "spiritual adviser" experience in Los Angeles. Instead I chose to follow my own school of psychology, the School of Repression.

In the School of Repression, one works to encourage the mind's ability to hide information from the conscience. Destructive behaviors occur when negative thoughts are not fully repressed. Psychoanalysis will only further expose this negativity. We argue that things are hidden for a reason and unearthing them only leads to unhappiness. It is not in one's best interest to be unhappy. Repression can help one trample any memory: like going to a Hungarian bathhouse and being forced to wear a very Eastern bloc, pink and brown rubber-lined bathing suit and matching cap while her own, stylish, navy blue Adrienne Vittadini suit hung in a nearby locker. It might help you mentally heal from a lye-soap flaying that was marketed as an exfoliating massage, and having that pink, rubber bathing suit stripped off in one stroke and two stumpy thumbs plugged into your rectum on the return stroke. I might also use repression to forget the hours I spent shivering with open pores and wet hair waiting outside for my lame-ass friends in not-so-balmy mid-December Budapest. And I could, perhaps more successfully, repress my lymphedema issues and put the sleeve away without further angst. I would waste no time exploring my motives for the decision or obsessing about any other seemingly hideous things that would reveal themselves in their own time.

Sunday morning, my last day in the hospital, Dr. Ree swung by to change my dressing. She had on yoga clothes and a backpack and looked about sixteen years old. She seemed very nervous and kept touching my shoulder. "Are you ready to do this?"

"Hell yeah!" I loved stitches ever since I was a kid and my father taught me how to take out my cats'. "Let's get a mirror!"

"Are you sure, Meredith? Sometimes people get upset."

"Whatever. There's a mirror in here." I led her into the little bathroom. She unswaddled my rib cage slowly. Finally, there it was. On the left side sat my smashed flat, deflated boob, and on the right side, nothing, just a thin line of steri-strip tape over the actual incision. Flat as a wall. There were no black stitches, no gruesome scar. It was just gone.

"You are a freaking magician! I so should have gone to medical school." I looked at it from every angle.

Thibault had been lingering in the background but I pulled him in front of the mirror. "Look," I said. He looked perplexed, like it was some sort of smoke-and-mirrors trick.

We were both expecting a horror show, bear mauling, or something. But this was so tidy that it was hard to believe a breast had ever been there. Then she wrapped me back up and left. I was officially eligible to join the Amazon archery club.

chapter twenty

When the breast was removed, skin from the surrounding area was pulled in and sewn over the exposed chest wall. Because my cancer had spread to the skin, more skin than usual, with a generous margin, was removed. It took a while for the stretched skin to reattach to the flesh in its new location. To aid healing, bandages were wrapped tightly around my rib cage to keep the skin and flesh in contact and to discourage the buildup of fluid in the area.

It didn't work. Serous fluid, a pale pink liquid, started pooling inside and making huge blisterlike pockets that jiggled when I poked them, which was constantly. Dr. Ree saw me immediately, probably because I called her, ranting hysterically about pus from a waffle-iron burn on my arm exploding on Erin Banks during dodge ball in seventh grade. Erin couldn't shut up about it for days and kept harping about how I'd ruined her stupid burgundy Member's Only jacket.

When Dr. Ree did see it, she rolled her eyes. She'd expected much worse. Often, she said, people wait until there is a liter or more of fluid before they call. So much fluid accumulates that it looks like the breast has grown back.

"What kind of crazy-ass lets that happen?" My blister thing was about four inches long by one inch wide and raised about half an inch and I couldn't bear the sight of it.

"I'll drain it. It'll only take a second and won't even hurt."

"You're going to what?"

"I'll just put a syringe into the incision here, where it's numb, and drain out the fluid."

I must have misheard her. She could not actually intend to stick a needle into the freshly healing cut from the surgery? But she did, four times, and each time she filled a big, fat reservoir full of cirrus. The girl who previously enjoyed rhinoscopy videos and fancied herself a rich, urban Moyle in her next life, almost blacked out. I could no longer brag about my unsqueamishness.

What was left of my chest, my lone boob, served no purpose whatsoever but presented plenty of problems. If I wanted to appear presentable, I was forced to wear a falsie.

The first falsie I got while healing from surgery was just a little cotton bag filled with stuffing. It was designed to fill in my chest, but not put too much pressure on the chest wall. The problem was that it had no weight to it and floated all over my shirt. I found it meandering about my torso, causing unsightly bulges. Once it even migrated above my real boob, forming a nice row of teats like you might see on a nursing sow. Thibault gently nudged it back into place, saying, "You are too *boo-ti-ful* to have the breasts of a farm beast."

The second falsie I got was called a prosthetic and had to be fitted professionally. It was made out of a mystery gel and designed to fill in the hollow parts under my arm as well as the breast and cleavage area. Seeing it made me realize just how much tissue the doctor had removed—a big chunk of my flesh was sitting on a shelf somewhere waiting for its place in the

St. Meredith reliquary, in a jar next to goiters and those weird cysts made of teeth and hair from undeveloped twins. Or worse, it was sizzling in the bottom of an incinerator. My little nipple, the same one I'd taken with me everywhere, off experiencing adventures of its own, no longer a passenger, but its own pilot.

The woman who fitted my prosthetic was a lovely older lady with an English accent working in a brazier and corset shop straight out of 1952. She gave me a bra to use for the fitting. This was unlike any bra I'd ever worn. It was from the days when maxi-pads had belts. It was enormous, of course, with two-inch-wide straps, underwire, total cup coverage, and a back band wide enough for three rows of four hooks. This was a middle school boy's worst nightmare. It looked like it was designed not only for breast support, but as a straitjacket and rib splint as well.

I'd seen a bra like that once before on the French equivalent of the Discovery Channel. It was a documentary about a tribal wedding in an African village. The bride had on the traditional grass skirt, copper jewelry, and animal-skin headdress. She also sported a stark white Maidenform bra much like the one I was wearing. Where she got it was unknown, but I figured it was donated by some seventy-year-old Lutheran missionary unable to bear the sight of the damage gravity, childbearing, and excessive sun exposure had done to unsupported breasts.

The bra brought tears to my eyes. Done were my cute little pink and orange leopard print demicups with spaghetti straps and diaphanous lace. The doctor had told me they were taking away my boob, not my lingerie. My tortured face must have said it all because the corset shop lady quickly scrambled and found something considerably less matronly. The new prosthetic looked quite natural and, except for misplacing it occasionally, caused me no aggravation at all. Plus, when I took it away, my washboard-like rib cage created a sveltness I found alluring. Many nights I fell asleep caressing the childlike boniness like it was some affection-craving, hairless cat.

It was late September and Northern California Indian summer was in full swing. It was the first time since treatment began that I didn't feel exhausted; I felt like swimming, a strange idea for me, not being a swimmer. I knew how to swim, even felt confident in the water, but I'd never taken to the whole swimming-as-a-sport thing, like doing laps and competing. In fact, the only time I had done that, not long after college, during my very brief membership at the YMCA, it had been really unpleasant.

First I had to get to the pool from the locker room. That required rinsing off in the group shower and witnessing a fat lady pull up her belly rolls to shave her pubic hair and then sudsing her bits so thoroughly I thought maybe the health department was coming to do a white-glove inspection. Another woman and her small daughter sat naked on the bare floor clipping their toenails.

Once in the pool area I tried to get into the pool without drawing any attention to myself. The problem was my suit; it was metallic and sporty and made me look like I should either be a barracuda or swim like one. I slipped into the lane closest to the locker room, put on my goggles, and tried to remember what my perverted summer camp counselor—the one who let his balls hang out of his shorts—always coached: keep your head down and splashing to a minimum.

So I swam a few laps and got some powerful cramps, but I kept going until I noticed this elderly gentleman wearing vintage, hip-hugging trunks, yellow with a brown belt and tortoiseshell buckle, watching me from the end of the lane. As I prepared to do my turn he tapped me on the shoulder and said, "Excuse me, but what is the agenda with your legs?"

" 'Cuse me?"

"Well, are you swimming or walking? I saw you from over there."

I stared at the guy for a good ten seconds. Finally he said, "Well, I'll let you get back to it," and walked away.

Was I walking or swimming? I continued my laps, trying to put him out of my mind. He certainly was a ballsy old goat, using some old-timey pickup line on me. That was when I noticed my own feet, almost directly below me. I wasn't gliding across the surface like some sexy water snake, attracting the attention of frisky old men, I was marching through it, almost perfectly upright, and my arms were spinning like two rusty pinwheels. Oh my God! Was it true that black people can't float? I always thought we historically didn't swim because if they thought we could, white people would have made us pull barges or something.

I tried to correct my position, but my feet kept sinking down, like they were made of lead. I arched my back, but then my belly would meander ahead of me. I tried the backstroke, but I was still perpendicular to the surface, only now I couldn't see where I was going. I was a goddamned swim-walking ethnic stereotype.

I sidestroked to the edge of the pool and climbed out. My flip-flops were waiting for me a few yards away and I stepped into them and headed toward the showers but quickly redirected myself when I glimpsed a woman flossing her teeth and spitting the findings onto the floor.

I thought the steam room would be better and, in fact, did enjoy a few minutes of solitude before I was joined by a portly nude woman. Before entering the steam room I had taken three clean towels from the shelf outside. One was wrapped around me, and the other two were under me, protecting my skin and orifices from the wet, ceramic bench. I didn't even want to think of the variety of germs on those tiles, basking in the moisture and heat.

The naked woman sat down on the dripping bench and scooched her ass around as if trying to form a nice suction. Soon another woman came in and the portly lady made room for her on the bench. But instead of standing up, moving down a step or two, like a normal person with even a vague belief in scientific discovery since the 1700s, she just smeared her buttocks along the ceramic seat, making a high-pitched squeaking squeegee noise followed by the fartlike skidding sound your wipers make when the windshield is dry. Then she giggled and said, "That wasn't too dainty, was it?"

I fled the steam room, dropped my left flip-flop on the way out, and had to hop on one foot all the way to my locker. There, I suffered through a woman plucking her armpit hairs while I dressed as quickly as possible and gathered my things.

Ten years had passed and I hadn't once had the desire to swim laps since that day. But suddenly, after months of abusing my body in the name of saving it, strapped to IVs, stuffed into giant X-ray machines, cutting it away piece by piece, this image of pulling myself through the cool, clear water, prisms in my eyelashes, and the refreshed feeling of stepping out into the bright sunshine was so appealing that I put on my suit and walked over to Karen's pool. It was beautiful with the waterfall running, but didn't fit the image I had in my head. There was too much shade and it wasn't big enough to swim proper laps. Plus, the bottom was painted dark indigo blue, not the crystal turquoise I wanted. I had to go to the community pool down the road.

I avoided all the hygiene sand traps of a public locker room by arriving prepared, suited up and rinsed off. The water was the ideal temperature and the sky and pool were perfect, matching shades of blue. I hopped into the slow lane and submerged myself, eyes open, goggleless, like they do on television, but never in real life because in real life "chlorinated water" is just code for diluted hydrochloric acid. My eyes started to sting and I found myself physically incapable of opening them; my lids locked down. But I pushed off anyway, unwilling to give up so quickly.

Something else immediately felt wrong. My right arm was not cooperating. Standing upright, since the surgery, my right arm wouldn't extend above the shoulder. It didn't seem to be muscle weakness, or tight tendons, but as though the joint had been refashioned and blocked. My range of motion was so limited, I couldn't lift my arm out of the water. It took me thirty gimpy stroke . . . drag . . . stroke . . . drags to get only halfway across the pool and I'd swum blindly into the lane dividers multiple times. I was out of breath, swallowing water, and embarrassing myself. I wiped my eyes, which felt better now that the tearing had begun, and turned back, hoping to reach the edge by doing the breaststroke. That is when I swam into a blurry mass of tawny-colored silicone, a nippleless blob bobbing like a big cow patty in the water. My falsie. I stuffed it back into my suit, frantically dog-paddled across two lanes to the edge, got out of the water, and drove home soaking wet. I did not need a more obvious sign that seeing Lucas grow up was not something I'd earn by overexerting myself, be it swimming or pedaling all over Tarnation. Lance Armstrong and I would find different paths.

chapter twenty-one

My vision started to abandon me somewhere along the way. It wasn't a specific event or time, but gradually, after starting chemotherapy, things just got darker and darker. I don't even remember when I bought extra lights or trimmed the trees to let in more sunlight, or when my face started aching from the squinting. My sister just said to me, not long after the mastectomy, that coming into my house was like entering an interrogation room.

Soon after that things started to blur. Reading was no longer an option, no matter how many watts bathed the page. The television was an amorphous blob of colors. The road was a guessing game; should I follow the streaks of light or avoid them? All I could do was practice the Braille sheets I ordered from the Lighthouse for the Blind, and hope Lucas wouldn't object to wearing a Seeing Eye dog harness.

Of course Dr. Yuen thought it was a brain tumor. She got me a CAT scan before I even finished explaining the symptoms. "Darkness!? Freaky. You gotta motor over to nuclear imaging." It wasn't, but I could add barium and radioactive isotope #7 to the growing list of toxins stored in my subcutaneous fat.

We finally decided that after a lifetime of hawklike vision I just might need glasses. I went to see the ophthalmologist. She gave me an eye test, telling me to guess the letters I could not see. "How, exactly," I asked, "will cheating on an eye exam help me?" After failing to read the first line she told me that my vision was 20/20. Had they changed the grading system? "I couldn't read even one letter."

"You can do everything you need to do," she said chipperly.

At this point Thibault physically restrained me from slapping the phantom head floating just next to her own, but my lunge still managed to wipe the smiles off her faces. She backed out of the room and a different, extremely professional and competent doctor fitted me for glasses.

That night at my parents' house, still upset by the shitty doctor's disregard, I interrupted my father's shredding to tell him what had happened. He shrugged and said, "I'd rather be dead than blind."

Sometimes, in elementary school, I got off the bus to buy candy at the Freeway Variety convenience store and would have to walk the last mile home. But instead of walking normally, I limped along with one leg rigid, as though it were wooden. Every now and then I stopped and pretended to adjust my fake limb, rubbing the painful stump, just above the knee, before marching on. When cars passed I wiped my brow and smiled courageously at the drivers. Sometimes they stopped and asked me if I needed help. I always said, "No, it's just a few more blocks. My mom would pick me up but she has to take my twin sisters to gymnastics. They're going to be the next Nadia Comaneci and Olga Korbut."

My delivery was so bad that most people just rolled their eyes and drove away. But every now and then the driver became overwhelmed with sympathy for the singleton, one-legged sister of twin world-class athletes, neglected by her mother and left to hobble home on her ill-fitting prosthesis, that I got the brave nod, the supportive, affirming smile given to Special Olympians when they run the hundred-yard dash in eleven minutes.

Blind people often complain that strangers touch them too much. They are always resting their hands on blind people's shoulders or hugging them in crosswalks. It startles them, is inappropriate, and disrespectful of boundaries. But touching is how you brave nod to a blind person. They can't see the tilted head, sad eyes, and condescending smile awarded to the sighted handicapped, the becrippled, and often, the cancerous.

I had been getting that smile from people who thought having cancer and raising a toddler was something heroic. And I liked it because it let me actually pretend to be heroic. But if I went blind, I wouldn't get the nods, I'd get the pats on the shoulder and the violated private space. People would treat me like a dog tied to a parking meter, feeling free to pet and caress it without invitation.

How soundly could I beat a transgressor with one of those flimsy canes? Would I even have the will to protect myself? Or would I be so overwhelmed by the darkness that my entire personality would alter and I'd cower under the caresses? I doubted it. People are who they are. Personalities don't change, just circumstances. It is my firm belief that adversity only strips the insulation from the foundation. If the foundation is weak, corrupt, or solid, its nature is simply revealed. Few situations are so harrowing as to build or deplete character. You either have it, or you don't.

The week I started radiation Thibault flew back to France for work. We'd been living for six months off our meager savings and friends' outrageous generosity. Wah, my college roommate, raised money for us by running the Boston Marathon in god-awful heat. Rebecca gave us her car. Karen let us live at her house. People made us disasteroles. My parents and in-laws hid bills from us on two continents. Knowing I would eventually reciprocate or die made it easy for me to accept the gifts graciously. Thibault, on the other hand, felt humiliated. It was his job to support his family. After five humbling months living off charity, Thibault couldn't stand it anymore. He took the only decent job he could find, a consulting gig outside Paris. That left me with Lucas and two daily radiation appointments for the next six weeks. From the degree of slumpiness in Thibault's shoulders as he mumbled good-bye at the airport, you'd have thought he was leaving me naked in the cold with a pack of wild dogs.

This was just the kick I needed to get out of the bed, out of the house, and out of the garden. I couldn't lounge around all day when I had to deliver Lucas to day care and be at the radiation clinic by eight-thirty. Once I was up and out I might as well stay out, so I went to the library and started working on the book I'd always promised my grandmother I'd write. I wrote every day between my appointments, then picked up the boy and took him home. I cooked dinner, gave my son a bath, and collapsed, like my legs had been chopped off, in bed by seven o'clock.

Even though my days were organized around my cancer treatment, and I still had all the physical trappings of a cancer patient, I felt normal again. I was only slightly sentient of mortality, and mostly only when other people awkwardly avoided using the word *death* around me. I didn't float on a parallel plane or get stuck in a purgatory-like existence, like some other patients I met. Perhaps it was the people around them that made melancholy possible. I had a small child who didn't give a shit who was sick or who was out of town; he wanted salami and string cheese NOW. With Thibault gone there was nobody around to appreciate any dramatic displays of moroseness.

One man told me, as he sat in the radiation waiting room working on the jigsaw puzzle, that his wife cried every single day as he drove her home from the appointment. I figured she must be stage IV with only weeks to live and was leaving behind young children and a fabulous career. To my surprise he said that she was childless, had stage I breast cancer, and had opted for a full and thoroughly unnecessary mastectomy when a lumpectomy would have been sufficient. Her doctors felt convinced that her cancer was gone and she would live to be an old woman.

"Why the Hell is she crying every day?" I asked.

He just rolled his eyes and said he suspected she had always cried every day; he just hadn't been there to witness it.

"Plus," he said, "she is milking the cancer thing. It legitimizes all of her maudlin emotions." It sucked because two days before she was diagnosed he told her he would leave if she didn't start antidepressants. Now she refused, claiming that she didn't want to add any more toxins to her body. Consequently, he was stuck with this emotional wreck and thought he'd lose all his friends and end up in Hell if he divorced her in the middle of this. So each day he left work and drove her to her radiation appointment. He sat and worked on the puzzle in the waiting room and then escorted her home, trying to block out her sobbing by singing over the Top 40 songs blaring on the radio.

"It would be one thing if she really had something bad," he mused. "But the fact is that nobody believes this disease really threatens her life. Heck, maybe she's just crying from disappointment."

When she came out after her appointment the husband looked irritated that he was being pulled away from his puzzle. It was actually a good one this time, a 3-D holograph of a coral reef. He knew he'd probably never see it finished. Most thousand-piece puzzles only lasted a day or two, and unless that freak who always stole one piece so that only he or she could experience the satisfaction of slipping that last tile into place wasn't due back until late the next day, the finished product would be long gone. He took a sentimental look at his handiwork, a deep breath, gave his wife an apologetic smile, and walked out the door with his hand placed gently on the small of her back.

His candor was unsettling. Who was I, for chrissakes? Not his therapist. For all he knew, I had the same "noncancer" as his wife. Maybe I was just as weird as she was. I could easily have been offended by his story. But my reaction seemed to be the least of his worries. He was just being honest and didn't seem either strained or relieved by the effort.

He seemed like the kind of guy who would kill that woman

in an utterly passionless moment. He'd hold her head under the bathwater while he gently scrubbed her back with a loofah. He'd hold it with incredible strength and apparent effortlessness until she stopped resisting. Then he'd dry himself off with one of the pink towels he never thought he'd own, call the police, and turn himself in. When they arrived, he'd be sitting in the living room, drinking beer from a chilled glass, while his wife lay slumped over, facedown in the tub.

Either that or he'd take care of her, never complaining, for the next thirty years—and fill his quiet moments with fantasies of drowning her. It was the worst kind of marriage. As I watched them pull out of the parking lot, I saw her study her reflection in the mirrored windows of the clinic and light a cigarette. She clearly wasn't concerned about the toxin called tar.

She was the bad-bride version of a cancer patient, a spoiled, insecure person who got away with being obnoxious because "it's her special day." Somewhere along the way she abandoned her belief in community: that death, even her death, was happening to all of us. She was exactly the kind of person I prayed never to reveal in myself. Nothing is less tolerable, more mockworthy or insulting, than self-indulgent hopelessness.

chapter twenty-two

It was still Indian summer, and six months had passed since my initial diagnosis. There was no evidence of disease and I was finished with treatment. My hair was growing back. We had some money. I could be something besides a cancer patient. Rebecca and Sandra, my palm-reading friend, threw a party for me, a barbecue to celebrate the end of it. They got a chocolate cake that said "Meredith Kills Cancer Dead" in big, pink, cursive letters and gave me presents like it was my birthday.

At one point I pulled Dr. Green, my radiation oncologist, away from the grill and into the house. "Hey," he said, "I spoke about you to this guy. He had some interesting ideas. You should talk to him."

"You have to see this first." I dragged him into the bathroom and he looked around, like there was some light fixture I thought he should buy for his new house or something. "What are you looking at? I want to show you my chest. It's disgusting."

He expected to see the burned skin he'd exposed to six weeks of intensive radiation. What he saw instead was that dead, blackened, charred tortilla-like skin after it had been soaked in chlorine water, then bandaged and unable to air out for a week.

"Ah!" escaped and he covered his mouth.

"Gnarly, eh?" I said proudly.

"What did you? How did you?" he stammered, eyes glued to the oozing, raw pink and pitch-black mess.

"I went swimming at the community pool. Well, kind of. It didn't really work out."

He recoiled, as if the gruesomeness might be contagious. "I guess not," he said, then we laughed. It was a reaction he would never have had in his professional white lab coat. But in his yellow polo shirt and swim trunks he was just a guy, my friend with the crazy X-ray machine. Everybody at the party was my friend and finally relaxed because I wasn't dying anymore. We barbecued meat and everybody rubbed my downy head. The party was meant to mark the official end of treating me differently. Instead of a sparklers show, perhaps we could punctuate the celebration with the long-overdue ass-kicking promised by my sister.

I hadn't exactly survived cancer yet—it was much too soon to claim that—but I had survived sixteen weeks of accelerated, dose-dense chemotherapy, a mastectomy, and fifty-four radiation appointments. My shot veins and maimed, scarred, and burned chest were battle wounds; the stubble on my head made me look like G.I. Jane. I felt like a war hero, but something about this didn't feel like a victory party. I was a soldier going into retirement; this was a retirement party.

At the end I gave a lame speech. I don't even remember what I said, but I cried right in the middle of my list of thank-yous. I grabbed Lucas and hid behind him and everybody was relieved to see me emotional finally about living or dying or not dying or losing my fancy Paris apartment, or whatever had just happened over the last six months.

Across the patio, Thibault caught my eye. He'd only been back from France for a few days, but already that freshness he'd had when he deboarded the plane had begun to wilt. It was as though my mere proximity drained him, although he'd never admit it, even to himself. His face looked sunburned and his shoulders slumped and he looked so exhausted that you'd have thought he had cancer.

It was much harder being the person taking care of the person with cancer. I got dibs on rest and pity and kindness and he got whatever crumbs were left over . . . after Lucas raked through them. This day should have marked the end of Thibault's indentured servitude, a chance to rejoice, but I'd only seen halfhearted smiles and polite laughter.

He paced himself emotionally for six months, just long enough to get us through the standard treatment, but now he knew it hadn't been enough. Despite my looking more normal and our publicly announcing that everything was finished, both of us sensed this party was not what it claimed to be. It was a way for our friends to gracefully dismount the Meredith Pink Ribbon Wagon, but as a celebration it was bogus and, at best, grossly premature.

The following week I went to see the doctor Dr. Green had mentioned in the bathroom at my party. Dr. Stone had lots of experience with my rare form of breast cancer and felt he could be helpful. What was one more doctor's appointment to me?

Dr. Stone studied my chart, examined me, and estimated my chance of recurrence somewhere around 80 percent.

"Eighteen? How exact! Not fifteen or twenty? Eighteen."

"Eighty."

"But it was only sixty percent when I started!"

"Survival averages were sixty percent. Recurrence is almost guaranteed." I was too stunned to respond. Semantics? It wasn't possible.

He suggested more chemotherapy, this time paired with a monoclonal antibody called Herceptin. I needed chemo every day for two weeks, then a week off before the Herceptin infusion, for an entire year, seventeen cycles.

This disease was going to be harder to shake than my three-boyfriends-ago boyfriend, Sean. It had only taken me a year to get rid of him and his ridiculous tantrums. In one typical fit he smeared a falafel into my dashboard because I said his new cologne smelled just a little bit like beef jerky. Then, when I told him he'd better clean it up he screamed, "Clean it yourself, and the rest of the shit in this frowzy hoopty!"

Frowzy hoopty? I couldn't date a man who'd pair those two words, who'd even use *frowzy*. "Frowzy? Frowzy hoopty?" Then I started laughing so he jumped out of the car at a stop sign.

I tried to break up with him after every tantrum, but once he realized what I was doing he just took his shirt off and confused me. I saw that chiseled, tan chest, like something from an underwear box, and completely lost my train of thought.

It was Rebecca's idea that I break up with him somewhere he couldn't undress, so we went to a restaurant. I told him it was over. After a minute of desperately tugging at his shirt cuffs, I suppose, expecting his clothing to become miraculously invisible, he rose and left me with the bill.

A month passed without a word and then he called to tell me he was at the airport, on his way to Europe. I was not particularly warm, but amicable, and wished him a safe trip. Before I could hang up he promised to call me during his layover in New York. When I sputtered a puzzled "What for?" he said only that his plane was boarding and that he had to go. I remember looking at the receiver as I hung it up, wondering if he had meant to call me or someone who cared.

About six hours later, just as I had almost forgotten the entire incident, the phone rang again: "Hi, babe, I'm in New York. I'll see Paul tonight and leave for Europe in the morning. He says hi." All I could muster up, being thoroughly discomposed, was: "Hi . . . Paul." Whoever that was. And how come he's calling me *babe*?

During his three-week trip he called me six times. Each time I stood dumbfounded, wondering if it was he or I who was completely deranged. The final call came from Denver. He was only two hours away and wanted to know if I could pick him up from the airport. "No fucking way," I should have said. "That is too girlfriendy and I'm not your goddamned girlfriend." Instead I stuttered through some lame story about going to sushi at Uzen with Rebecca and the girls and that he should have called me sooner.

Just as I was recounting the story Sean showed up at the restaurant, full of smiles and holding a bag full of little gifts for me. He actually held my hand at the table and managed to completely disregard the dropped jaws and dumbfounded stares. He had simply chosen to ignore the fact that we were all utterly appalled by his presence.

He paid for my dinner and as we were leaving said, quite loudly, "I'll follow you to your apartment, or we can go to mine if you prefer." After realizing that I was paralyzed by bafflement, and hence unable to respond, Rebecca stepped in and informed us both that I would not be going to his apartment. He squeezed me and said cheerily, "Fine then, yours it is." Then bolted down the street before Rebecca could rebut.

Sean beat me home and sat waiting, shirtless, on the stoop, rhapsodizing about the balmy warm night and how good the air felt. The night was neither balmy nor warm and goose bumps covered his skin, but still, the entire speech I'd prepared on the way home was instantly deleted from my memory.

He kept me distracted for almost three days. Then I said his friend Blas had a nondescript name and Sean smashed my butter dish, the only thing I salvaged from my Spanish car accident. We were back to the same old cycle and I could only reminisce fondly about that carefree month when I thought I was free.

I guess Dr. Stone saw the discontent on my face because he jumped to reassure me that these nearly fifteen hundred pills, over a pound and a half of poison, wasn't a big deal. Xeloda, the chemotherapy, was really easy, and oral, no pricks or pain, and then just seventeen infusions. But the nature of the next stage was neither here nor there; I was lamenting the brevity of the pause. They told me I'd have chemo, mastectomy, and radiation, and then I'd be done. What was all that? The standard treatment. Anything more, like another year of chemo, would be experimental. I guess I should have been grateful, but we weren't allowed even a full week before getting roped back into the drama and drudgery of Meredith having cancer.

There was no time to waste moping because I had serious issues to resolve before continuing treatment. How was I supposed to take seventeen more infusions? My veins were already so decimated by the chemo that even drawing blood from them without putting a needle deep into the center of my forearm was impossible. I needed a port—another surgery, but no big deal, a procedure so easy they let radiologists do it. No worries. The only person to pipe up was Dr. Yuen, who exclaimed, "That's like totally crazy! A year of Xeloda! As if!"

I remembered a girl who lived on my floor senior year of college. She was telling another girl that she could treat a yeast infection with acidophilus yogurt. The infected girl denied being desperate enough to put Yoplait in her vagina just yet and the other girl said, "Give it enough time and you'll put your grandpa's dentures up there if it would help." I didn't want to get to that point. A year of "no big deal" sounded good to me, especially since I'd gotten that 80 percent number. So I signed up for port surgery, scheduled my first infusion for a few weeks after that, and pretended like this was cool. Two weeks later, three weeks after my barbecue, I was back on the operating table.

chapter twenty-three

When I learned how many people came to wait in the hospital during my mastectomy surgery I felt ambivalent. Although a clear indication of their love, I did not think it was especially helpful to me personally at the time, with my being unconscious and all. I also felt slightly obligated to write thank-you cards, a task that I considered a chore. And I may have had lingering guilt over not writing those cards, which was also not helpful.

Since my big Meredith Kills Cancer Dead party supposedly meant that my friends and family could dedicate themselves to other causes (and to avoid any guilt over unsent thank-you cards), I did not tell anyone extra when my port surgery was scheduled, or that I was even having another surgery at all. I tried to drive myself to the appointment, but my keys mysteriously disappeared and Thibault, who was conveniently between clients, drove me.

It was a really sunny, beautiful day and I just did not want to spend it at the hospital. Other people were in their cars bouncing to music, or smiling and chatting; and I was a tense little ball of angry resistance. Of all the hospital visits, this was the first one where I felt put-upon, like I'd been chosen unjustly to suffer through this.

Thibault started to turn into the parking lot.

"Just drop me here," I said.

"I'll meet you inside."

"Just drop me off."

"I'm coming with you."

"If you come inside I will bite off my tongue."

"What does that mean?"

"It means that I will push my teeth through my tongue until it is in two pieces."

"Then you won't be able to talk, right?"

"I wanna go alone! Shit. Unlock the door. What am I? A fucking hostage?" It was my first nonsteroidal temper tantrum. He unlocked the door, blew me a kiss—which I smashed violently between my palms—and drove off. I waited at the corner to make sure he didn't just circle the block and then park in the lot.

The radiology department kept me waiting for two hours in a room with people who just needed X-rays. These people were allowed to eat any delicious-smelling junk food they wanted, as they weren't getting anesthesia. They also felt relaxed and annoyingly chatty, as they weren't getting SURGERY!

I sat in my chair, fuming. Hadn't I done every goddamned thing I was supposed to do? And done it with a smile? When would this shit be over? I marched up to the counter.

"My life expectancy is less than eighteen months. I'm not wasting any more time in this stupid waiting room. Tell the doctor I left."

I headed for the door, then turned around and went back to the counter.

"Meredith Norton. Can you tell the doctor now that Meredith Norton is leaving? That Meredith Norton is not wasting any more time in this stupid waiting room?"

"You done with the drama?" My vision was impaired so what appeared to be an aged Filipino woman could have been my sister, but I didn't remember my sister saying she was getting a receptionist job at the hospital. "Sit down and let me go see what's happening. Just wait." I remained standing, arms crossed, on the verge of tears. "Come with me. We'll ask together. Come on, girl."

She led me down a corridor and tapped on a windowless door. When she peeked inside I saw the nurses in almost total darkness eating food off the operating table.

"We were just finishing up and coming to get her. Leave her here. Come in. Sit down. We'll just clean this up." They cleared away the mess, threw out their lunches, and tried to soothe my mood to no avail. Finally, they stopped talking to me entirely, not even asking me to remove my necklace or earrings, just gently doing it themselves.

What did I have to be so pissed off about? And why was I choosing these strangers to unleash on? I put on the gown, lay on the table, and they were about to administer the anesthesia when I snapped.

"Who is this mysterious doctor who is supposed to OPER-ATE on what's LEFT of my BODY?!"

"Dr. Sheinbaum?"

"Is he the one using a KNIFE to CUT into an artery near my HEART?"

"I hope not."

"What!? I'm SUPPOSED to get a PORT. I'm MEREDITH NORTON, in for a PORT!"

"We know who you are," she said patiently. "It is a VEIN, not an ARTERY."

Her mocking me was not appreciated. "I want to see the doctor NOW!"

Dr. Sheinbaum sat next to me on a little footstool that put his head at about my shoulder height, as I was lying down. He reminded me of the boyfriend I broke up with because he was too short, and looked like a child sitting at the grown-up table. It wasn't sexy then, and it wasn't confidence-inspiring now. But he answered my questions, which I managed to scream at him fluidly rather than in randomly accented little bursts, showed me the gadget—a Cook titanium Vital-Port Vascular Access System—and I gave up.

Resistance was futile, and I had no more energy left to fight or be strong or even care. This is what was happening. I would soon have yet another scar and a freakish, half-inch-high ridged lump the diameter of a quarter poking from under my clavicle. It was time to accept that my body was just junked up and unless I wanted to face dating with this monstrosity, I'd better start being nicer to Thibault.

Thankfully I fell asleep, had the surgery, and made it home somehow. I had no recollection of getting to my parents' house or into my sister's bed fully clothed—a habit that made Thibault crazy—or falling back asleep. I do remember waking up abruptly, however, much later, grabbing my left arm, clutching my chest, and shrieking, "Daddy! Daddy!" He left the televised football game on, which was blaring through the house, and rushed to my side, just as he had all those times I tried to pee fire after soaking for hours in Mr. Bubble bubble bath, a known irritant to the urinary tract.

"What's the matter with you?" he asked, perplexed, as if I'd spent the day counting money and petting a poodle on my yacht.

"Stabbing! Stabbing! My chest! Aaah! My arm. I can't breathe. Aah!" He reached to remove the bandage. It was so sensitive I screamed. He looked at me like I was some sort of talking fish.

"It's like squeezing! I'm going to faint. I'm going to vomit!" Those were heart attack symptoms. Even I knew that. He left the room. Was I actually dying, of a heart attack, at thirty-three? *Crise cardiaque* at *trente-trois*. It sounded like a foreign film.

I'd done it now. Why did I let a radiologist operate on me? Was this the culmination of a lifetime of poor choices, starting with taking that grape Kool-Aid up to my room when I was six years old? I had so many better options: drinking it downstairs in the kitchen with the linoleum floor, taking it up the maid's wooden stairs instead of the front stairs with the yellow, deep shag carpet, filling the cup only 80 percent instead of 101 percent so it could slosh around without tearing that delicate surface tension dome that peaked over the brim. Then, when I saw my three-year-old brother hanging over the railing from the upstairs landing, ten feet from smashing himself onto a Tiffany lamp, I wouldn't have gotten caught. I could have pulled him to safety with two hands and gone on my pointless little six-year-old way. Instead, I had to hold him with one hand and the Kool-Aid with the other, watching it spill drop by drop onto the carpet for the eons it took my mother to find and rescue us. She said I did the right thing, saving my brother over the rug, but my dog still got sent to a farm in Washington State. My mother swore the two things weren't related, that the Siberian husky was going crazy in our small backyard in blazing-hot California, but my tiny mind was unable to believe her. I didn't even believe the dog was on a farm. She'd put him to sleep because stupid Meredith had to have Kool-Aid in her bedroom.

It all happened right outside the room where I lay in my sister's bed. The rug was gone, replaced by a not-so-'70s, short-loop, cream-colored wool, but the memory lingered, nearly as unsettling as the pain in my chest.

"Are you getting morphine?" I cried hopefully toward the hallway.

A few moments later my father returned.

"Where have you been? I can't breathe!"

"Usually 'I can't breathe' means 'I can't speak.' Venous contractions."

I thought he said "penis contractions" and that made me laugh because I am immature.

"Penis contractions?"

"You got a port, not a penis. Venous contractions, Meredith, in the subclavian vein."

"What?"

"The subclavian vein is a thick vein, about the width of your finger, that joins with the jugular to form the superior vena cava, which enters the heart at the right atrium. Didn't your doctor tell you this?"

"I don't know. His chair was so low."

"What could that possibly have to do with anything?"

"It was distracting or something."

"Or something? I'm pleased to know you can be distracted, or something, from your surgery consult by the height of a man's chair."

"For the love of God, Daddy, just tell me, please."

"Well, he punctured the subclavian and inserted the line from the port. Probably about four or five inches rest inside the vein. The vein doesn't like it; it's irritating and causes little spasms."

"Spasms?"

"Yes, Meredith, what you are feeling are spasms, venous spasms, or contractions. They can be quite painful."

"You just looked that up?" I asked through clenched teeth, fighting off another spasm.

"What am I, a first-year anatomy student? No, it's almost the end of the third quarter; I went to check the score."

"No booby?" Lucas stood next to the bed holding his little palm up. Then he pushed a sippy cup toward me. "Want some? No booby? No booby?" The clear emphasis on the word *no* made it clear he thought I'd gotten another mastectomy.

"Come here, sugar." I reached out to help him up.

"Booby hurt." He stepped back, remembering the weeks after the mastectomy when any and all contact with my chest was off-limits. It was traumatic for him, my little snuggle maggot, not to be allowed to touch me. This time I'd just grin and bear it, and not put a ban on the hugs.

"It's okay." He leapt on me like that killer rabbit in *Monty Python*. I didn't even have time to block him, and he managed to land his full weight on the newly installed port. His scabby little knee ripped out the anchoring sutures that fixed the port to my chest wall and tore through the stitches that closed the wound.

"AYAHHHHHH!!!" I howled so savagely that Lucas jumped off the bed, ran, and hid. There was no panic in his departure, just urgent flight, the nonsuppressible instinct to flee. He took off so purposefully, skillfully, knees high and little arms pumping, that it made me think. At one and a half years old he'd just recently started to see me as someone separate from himself, not just a smoochy jug of milk who kept his ass clean. And that separate person was always recovering from something, sleeping, or screaming. This was the only Mommy he knew. It was horrible. I was actually ashamed.

I was too depressed to return to the hospital to get the port reattached so I just taped the wound closed with butterfly bandages and left the port to float around under the skin. Ultimately, my father assured me, the pocket would scar up and keep the disk from sliding about.

The heart-attack-mimicking venous contractions lasted for more than twenty-four hours and Lucas avoided me or cried in my presence for the better part of three days. My whole chest was sore from the inch-long incision and my mood was black. The port surgery was the first indication that this extra year of treatment would not be as effortless and ignorable as everyone, save prophetic Dr. Yuen, had said.

chapter twenty-four

The "super-easy-nothing-to-it" Xeloda chemo was misrepresented as well. There were up to six pills to take a day, three in the morning and three at night. They were huge, chalky horse pills that made me gag. According to my doctor, most people reported no side effects from Xeloda—and with the administration being oral, they were almost like vitamins. The constant attack on your body's cells went virtually unnoticed. Either my physiology differed greatly from every previous Xeloda patient's, or Xeloda patients were the most unobservant collection of people on Earth.

I don't know what about me would have expected a typical reaction; I'd never had a typical reaction to anything in my life. I'd found myself outside of the pack often enough that being surprised by it at this point would seem like a mental health issue.

When the San Francisco Museum of Modern Art first opened its new building in 1995 I flocked, like everybody else, to see it. They didn't have much of a collection at that point so I wandered from gallery to gallery utterly unimpressed by anything other than the architecture. Not being a big architecture person I wanted to leave, but Rebecca kept dragging me along until we finally reached the top floor. And that is where I saw it, the most sublimely tacky thing whose splendor I've ever been allowed to bask in: Jeff Koons's five-hundred-pound porcelain sculpture of Michael Jackson and his chimpanzee, Bubbles, the one he rescued from a research lab and then serenaded while recording the *Bad* album. The two sat on a bed of roses, Bubbles on his best friend's lap, in matching gold marching band uniforms. It was as if all the hideous perversity, shallowness, and emptiness of celebrity culture had been miraculously transmuted from folly into glazed china.

I shrieked in delight. The room full of unapproving artgoers spun around to see what fool was clapping and yelling, "Finally! God bless Jeff Koons!"

"You're kidding!" a woman who seemed way too old for her extra-short art-chick bangs asked me. "It's horrible. And it's awful. I'm embarrassed to be American." More people chimed in, eager to dissuade me from my adulation of this artwork and its creator. Their efforts were futile. I'd never been so awash in the gloss in my life. I felt like getting naked.

Rebecca must have seen it in my eyes because she pushed me toward the elevator and out of the building, only letting me stop briefly to buy postcards at the museum store. I got enough to put a picture of Michael and Bubbles in every place my eyes habitually lingered: my bathroom mirror, over the kitchen sink, on the television, on my steering wheel. Nearly everybody who saw it said, "Damn, that's ugly."

And I always responded wistfully, "We walk alone, Jeff. Genius needs only one friend." But when it came to my Xeloda treatment, I didn't need a friend; I needed someone who could tell me how to deal with these side effects supposedly nobody else ever experienced.

There were four problems with my treatment. One, the

pills made me sleep so heavily that Lucas took to peeling open my eyelids to wake me up. The phone, car alarms, fire alarms, shaking, and pinching failed to stir me. I even napped through Lucas' falling out of his bed. Thibault heard him shrieking hysterically from halfway down the driveway and ran into the house only to discover his son clutching my limp arm and screaming into my ear.

Two, the pills caused freakish skin discoloration. Usually, as winter neared, I lost pigment and turned yellower and yellower. With Xeloda, as December approached, I got blacker and blacker. At first I thought it was a tan, but when I tan I turn browner, with a tinge of red. This color was black. The sides of my tongue, my gums, and, once again, my palms grew darker and more dead-looking with every pill.

Three, aside from the aesthetic problem, my skin was terribly thin and paperlike and ripped on anything with an edge, no matter how dull. The nubby plastic antennae on my cordless phone punctured me several times. The edges of my calculator sliced through my skin like a samurai sword. I barely bled, though, as I was as desiccated as a mummy. The dry skin separated and could be peeled off in thick, rubbery patches. Andrea made the hour-long drive several times just to come peel giant swathes off my feet. She sat at the end of my bed, peeling and talking about her love life. "There's definite potential with this one," she'd say. "He's both a Pisces and a Prince fan!"

Thibault tried not to vomit, but secretly I knew he found the peeling and Andrea's eagerness to do it uncouth. And while he'd rub my aching feet with his bare hands, he used gardening gloves to pick up and dispose of the foot skin–covered paper towel I'd left on the bedside table.

These issues were masked by wearing Thibault's big shirts so I could hide and protect my blackened hands inside long sleeves. I opened my mouth only as wide as was absolutely necessary to stuff in food or mumble. It was like having braces with rubber bands all over again, only back then, the sharp snap of the elastic bands wasn't nearly as powerful for behavior modification as shame.

"Taste this." Thibault handed me a spoonful of the beef bourguignonne he'd been cooking for six hours. The whole house, even the yard, smelled like stew. I fed my hands up opposite sleeves, clear to the elbows. He frowned. "Do not *Popoie* my shirt, please."

"Popeye your shirt." I still didn't reach for the spoon.

He sighed and tried to feed me directly. My mouth only opened slightly, revealing neither gums nor tongue.

"You are not being serious!" he said, exasperated. I opened just a smidge more. "I will not support eating *dees ords*!"

"What?"

"Anorexie, bulimie?"

"Disorders," I mumbled.

"Stick out your tongue."

"Uh uh."

"Stick out your tongue and let me see."

"I look like a parrot," I whispered.

He pulled down gently on my chin. I stuck my tongue out at him meanly, petulantly. He kissed it before I could snatch it back.

The fourth, most debilitating chemotherapy side effect was peripheral neuropathy. The books explained it as numbness, tingling, a pricking sensation, sensitivity to touch, or muscle weakness in the extremities. It could be vague and intermittent, or intense and constant. In extreme cases it could lead to organ failure.

On a scale of 1 to 10, with 1 being vague and intermittent numbness and 10 being constant intense pain and organ failure, I rated myself around a 7. The sensation I lived with all the time was that feeling you have when you try to make a fist but your hands are asleep: that stinging, burning cramp that dissolves as your circulation recovers. Imagine if your circulation never recovered, for three months, day or night, asleep or awake, in both your hands and feet. There wasn't just sensitivity to touch, but hypersensitivity, as though the ground was either on fire, or a bed of nails, and every object was razor sharp.

A typical chore—let's say getting a bottle for Lucas—might look something like this: Meredith with a lopsided tangle of newly sprouted hair (wearing the pajamas Thibault put on me the night before last, but didn't have the chance to take off yesterday morning before leaving for work, so I wore them all day yesterday, then slept in them last night, and am wearing them all day today as well) crawling across the floor on my knees and elbows to the kitchen. Lucas, seeing this opportunity to ride me like a horse, climbs onto my back. Now, in order to keep him from falling, I must hold him with my elbows, shuffling exclusively on my knees.

Once I reach the kitchen and convince the eighteen-month-old on my back to dismount, I pull open the refrigerator door with my teeth. We've attached a handy towel that makes this possible. Then I grab the milk with my forearms and start to curse. Some Frenchman with full dexterity has folded closed the milk carton! I ask Lucas to help me, but he thinks it's funnier to put his fingers, all the way to the knuckle, up my nose. I can't swat them away because I'll drop the milk, ah, which I've just dropped anyway. He runs out the door and I have no choice but to get on my feet and chase him barefoot before he gets down the gravel driveway. Each step is agony. Each step brings tears to my eyes. Each cry makes Lucas think this game is funnier and funnier. Eventually, I stop chasing, crawl back to the house, and he follows, tired of the game and ready for his bottle.

After he falls asleep I lay down next to him. My feet feel like embers. They are actually throbbing. I decide to use meditation and exchange this feeling for another, more pleasant one. I think about my friend Joanna and the big confession she made to me once. She very sheepishly asked if I ever, when falling asleep, felt like I had really *beeg* (she's Australian) hands. Had I ever felt enormous hands floating at my sides?

"You know, in that fuzzy time between wake and sleep?"

"Somebody with big hands?" What was she talking about?

"No, your own *beeg* hands, like five or *seecks* feet long, just *flaytin'* weightlessly?"

I teased her relentlessly after that confession, and to this day think fondly of her whenever I see foam #1 fingers, but during the peripheral neuropathy period, I secretly coveted her disorder. *Beeg,* painlessly relaxed hands sounded awfully pleasant. I could use them to hold Lucas' tiny little tooth-brush, or my own fork. Then he wouldn't have tiny little cav-ities on his brand-new tiny little teeth and my husband wouldn't have to feed me like I was a stroke victim.

Hands and feet weren't so different. Tingling and stinging weren't so distinct. Warm and burning, throbbing and puls-ing, potato potahto. An hour of positive thinking had me back in the zone.

It was during this time that we decided to go back to France for a visit. There was no reason not to. I could be tired on any continent. Plus, I'd left Paris ten months earlier for a quick trip home to California. I'd even neglected to tell most people I was leaving; the trip was such a nothing thing. Next thing they heard we'd fled the country and I was dying and bald and losing my boobs. We decided to go for three weeks around Christmas. That way Lucas would have plenty of opportuni-ties to escape from me in the multilevel, ungated stairwell, marble floor, antique-filled baby death trap that is my in-laws' home and I'd have plenty of opportunities to look pitiful and incompetent and visit some friends.

The first week I locked myself in a room for several hours while the family went out. A draft blew the door closed in the room where I'd been planted in front of the television. Kneel-ing in front of the door, I pawed at the handle with the heel of my palms. There was no option of grasping it; my hands were so weak. Some days I just woke up paralyzed, but this day the weakness was due to overexertion. Earlier that morning, be-ing too ashamed to call Thibault with his whole family within earshot, I'd exhausted all my hand strength by holding toilet paper tightly enough to wipe my ass. When they returned, I was lying on the floor wearing shearling boots, the only thing that gave me any comfort, on my hands.

As I lay there waiting for them, I remembered Maceo, my high school heartthrob, telling me, during one of our many hours of virgin snuggling, that he would love me even if I were just a head. It seemed so romantic at the time, that he loved me so abstractly. But recently, my body had been so burdensome, failing so miserably, that I almost preferred to ditch it and just be a head.

I was fine lying on the ground, but Thibault and his two handsome brothers picked me up and spoon-fed me a tiny pot of yogurt and I felt better. Then they turned on the video console and I watched them play Burnout 3 until I fell asleep. I had no choice; I couldn't leave.

The second week we went down to the country house so Lucas could stare at the cows and delight the grandparents with his stubbornness. Thibault's aunt had arranged for me to get a Herceptin infusion nearby so I could stay on schedule. The doctor reviewed my chart, asked me a few questions, and gave me the infusion, fifteen hundred dollars' worth of drugs, free of charge. Then he very casually asked me what I was doing for my side effects.

"Complaining."

"No, really?" he asked.

"Really." I said. "I'm a complainer. And I've reduced my dosage from six to two pills a day."

"Less than that isn't even worth taking."

"So I've heard."

"But there are drugs for this." He looked at me suspiciously.

"My doctor said there are no drugs."

"That is nonsense."

"But my American doctor said there is no treatment for this. Why would he say that?"

"Do you want the drugs or not?"

"Hell, yes!" He gave me three pills. Then he recommended that I take vitamin B_6, 200 mg a day, until I finished chemotherapy. That would prevent any recurrence of peripheral neuropathy. Twelve hours later my hands and feet were fine. I have only once, ever, loved a Frenchman more, maybe not even as much, and I married that one.

chapter twenty-five

I caught a cold on the flight home from France. For two or three days it was nothing more than an annoyance; I fought it off successfully. Then, between the time I left my parents' house for dinner and arrived at my house an hour away, the germs either blitzkrieged me or my body exhausted its very last defense. I was shaking and dizzy and freezing and sweating and could barely drag Lucas into the house. Why was Thibault still in France?

I called Rebecca. She was hosting a dinner party, but without hesitation offered to be at my house in an hour, as quickly as it would take to drive there. In the interim she sent her sister, who lived much closer. Her sister had had a blood transfusion earlier that day but came and got my son anyway. I don't remember either one of them arriving, but later Rebecca told me that I looked like I had Ebola.

I lay in bed delirious, sicker than ever, literally too weak to walk, too weak to get water, too weak to go to the bathroom, shivering and sweating, closer to death than ever before. I had freaky dream sequences and a few semilucid moments when the idea of being hospitalized came to mind. I was dying from a common cold. This is what happened to Victorian women after they got rained on; they fell ill and succumbed. I should call someone. Thibault? A doctor? The phone was ringing. It was my mother saying I needed to get my son.

"I thought he was with Rebecca."

"He was. Now he's here. I have to get ready for my Thursday meeting." Thursday? Dinner was Sunday night. Solomon Grundy worse on Thursday . . . died on Friday. I hadn't peed for three days? I looked at my water bottle, still half-full. That explained no peeing. I looked at my clock radio; it said Tuesday. What!?

"Meredith, are you there?"

"Today is Tuesday."

"You need to come and get Lucas."

I stood up and saw that the knife I'd been dreaming was gutting me again and again was just my belt buckle. I pulled it out through the loops of my jeans and laid back down freshly exhausted.

"I'm sick, Ma. Call Rebecca."

"She has her own kids to take care of."

"Call Rebecca."

Several years ago my friend Sandra was reading my palm and remarked that one of the lines on my hand implied that I had strayed from my proper path. Doing so only brought on suffering. Sandra assured me that if I remedied my situation the lines would change. The palm is an evolving document. It reports the past, present, and future. But destiny is not engraved and the shifting lines would prove that.

At the time I was in the process of closing my design company, and hopefully putting an end to the biggest mistake of my life. For three years Rebecca and I owned Norton Whittaker, Inc. We ran the company like a sitcom episode, never doing work and wasting our time on hilarious, far-fetched distractions.

We made slutty Christmas calendars for our neighbors with our own faces digitally covering the half-nude model on the *Hot Rod* magazine cover. Months were spent battling rodent infestation, and although we certainly had the resources to replicate Mapliffer's solution, we found less effective, more time-consuming methods with which to waste our time. We built model villages, rearranged furniture obsessively, and bred chinchillas. I can honestly say we spent more time with our feng shui expert than with our sales rep.

But between the high jinks, Rebecca and I fought like Arabs and Jews. I will diplomatically say that our working styles did not mesh, but it was a fundamental difference between how we each viewed money that really caused the problems. Rebecca worked by the motto of "It takes money to make money." I thought that if we didn't have money, we shouldn't spend money.

"Rebecca, why do we have a million Post-its?" We were standing in front of the office supply shelf eating ramen noodles.

"Because I don't like the yellow ones so I got the neon ones and they were cheaper in bulk. We saved like two hundred dollars."

"How do you save two hundred dollars on something that only costs five dollars?"

"If you buy one package its like five dollars, but if you buy fifty it's only two dollars each. You save three bucks a package."

"But we don't need fifty goddamned packs of Post-its! And

the yellow ones are only a dollar a pack, and they have three times as many Post-its in a pack of yellow as in neon."

"But I don't like the yellow ones."

"Who fucking cares?! You spent what? Six times as much, times fifty, because you don't like yellow?!" I started throwing the Post-its in a box, ready to return them to the store. Then I noticed my fingers were all sticky.

"What is this"—sniffing—"mouse piss?"

Ring! Rebecca ran to answer the phone while I fumed at the ruined Post-its.

"Norton Whittaker . . . this is her."

"This is SHE, Goddamnit!!!!"

Apparently the mouse pissing on the Post-its thought I was screaming at him, not my partner, and attacked. It leapt off the shelf like a furry little bullet right into my hair.

Eventually the whole thing proved too much aggravation for Rebecca and she just stopped coming. She walked out one day and did not come back to work ever, or call, for two weeks. I spent the next six months working, trying to pay back our suppliers. Finally I admitted that despite my efforts I had exhausted all my resources, mental and otherwise. Rather than make things worse I decided to close shop and move on.

It was the first time since I was sixteen and went to Hawaii that ordinariness defined me. Nothing about Meredith was so special as to exempt me from failure. Swimming one day off the shores of Oahu it occurred to me that not only was there no land in sight, but I couldn't see the bottom of the crystal-clear ocean either. At least there were no sharks, I thought, just before a cloud of sand rose up, obscuring my legs. In the panic that overcame me I tried to climb out of the water, not onto anything, it was just me dog-paddling in the Pacific, but I tried to climb on top of the water, like Jesus. Quite surprisingly, it didn't work.

Several hours later, bobbing limply with disappointment in my lack of superpowers, exhausted and dehydrated, I was rescued by the Coast Guard. It must have been how I desperately clung to him, straddling his legs like a baby monkey, but the rescuer couldn't get me to stop burrowing my face in his groin. Then I started sobbing and wiping my snotty nose against his trunks and the other guards couldn't even resist laughing. One guy on deck said to the guy I was glued to, "You two know each other?" It ended up being so hilarious that I forgot how dreadful it felt not having superpowers. The funny ending instantly canceled out the not-being-able-to-walk-on-water disillusionment.

When I walked out of Norton Whittaker the last time, I was worse off than half drowned. My weight had dropped to under a hundred pounds, I was bankrupt, and I despised my best friend. I no longer felt exempt from the foibles of the ordinary woman. My adventures could, and did, end in disaster, not just some funny anecdotes. Norton Whittaker destroyed the optimist in me. It made me fearful and distrustful and hateful. In all seriousness, the overall experience was so traumatic that I'd welcome ten different kinds of cancer before I chose to relive losing that business.

Rebecca and I obviously restored our friendship and it's a good thing. Without her I'd have completely fallen apart. It took awhile, but I knew it would happen after she had the gall to bring me a present from her "retirement" trip to Venice, Italy. It was a tiny Venician glass poodle no bigger than a black-eyed pea. It was the biggest thing she could afford . . . after her trip to the Prada outlet. You have to love a girl who admits to that while you are stuck at home preparing personal bankruptcy papers.

chapter twenty-six

Thibault and I were trying to buy a used car after shame-lessly borrowing Rebecca's for nine months. I found one in the paper and called the woman to arrange a test drive. She lived near my parents. When I told her I knew the area well she said, "Oh, then you must know me. I'm the one with breast cancer." I replied, "Which one? Like, every third woman you meet has breast cancer."

From the front door of her house, she never let me inside. I saw that the walls were absolutely covered with framed pic-tures of herself and her family posed perfectly candidly. I later saw her Web site and in the images section she had every step of the cancer process documented: the tender hands of the nurse, the hair fallen on the floor, her daughter's small hands touching her bald head, the IV bag hanging from its hook. All the pictures were black-and-white and impeccable.

Seeing all her photographs made me feel like such a talent-less slacker, full of envy, like Jeff Conaway, the actor who played Bobby from *Taxi*, who grew to hate Tony Danza be-cause they'd started out together, but Tony took off and Jeff just floundered. I just felt lame and since my hair had come back and I could walk and I'd had my big I Whooped Cancer barbecue, that opportunity to exploit my situation and to enjoy the perks were over. I was a has-been—the worst kind—still working, still out there, still in treatment, only nobody knew.

A month before my diagnosis I went to an art exhibit at the Center for Japanese Culture in Paris. One of the installations was a computer terminal with the screen projected overhead. Simultaneously counting up and down were the life spans of the volunteers willing to input their data into the system. Several people refused to participate and I just looked at them like they were retarded. "What was the issue?" I thought as I typed my name and birthday. Immediately, the counter started to add up the seconds since my birth: one billion sixty-nine million, two hundred eighty-six thousand, four hundred one, two, three . . . fine. Next I had to project my death day. I picked a random day the year Lucas will turn fifty. That way I would be old enough to die, but Lucas wouldn't be so young that living off his inheritance would destroy his ambition.

The instant I hit RETURN my life started counting down. I had a billion five hundred seventy-six thousand, eight hundred and seven, six, five . . . seconds until my death. I couldn't undo it and didn't even want to. I would have forgotten about it completely were it not for all the people staring at me, pointing and whispering.

That night at dinner I had no appetite. The *chou farci* placed before me was taken away untouched. The caramel flan sat like a lump of gelatinous dead flesh on a dessert plate. All I could think of were those people, and how their reaction was forcing me to think about that damnable counter speedily unwinding my life, chipping away, second by second, even while I slept, like waves on the beach. Why had it taken me four hours to understand how unsettling the concept was? It was a museum, filled with artwork meant to be provocative.

Everybody else perfectly understood that recording your death day was nothing if not horribly creepy. With this cancer experience, had I again missed the significance until it was too late? They were cowards?! Ha! I was a fool!

No matter how unique people seem, they can always be grouped into categories: fools and cowards, tops and bottoms, wolves and sheep, as was proven in a sixth grade science fair experiment by one of my classmates. Sage Edwards was one of those painfully, socially destructive middle school nerds who would probably become a billionaire by thirty and marry a talentless, but wildly attractive, B-level actress.

His theory was that when people experience something traumatic, they compound the problem by purposely introducing more trauma to themselves. He built a fish tank and filled it with creatures well known for their strikingly humanlike behavior patterns: guppies. In one corner of the tank was a little cage stuffed with feeding pellets; in the other corner a blinking strobe light and a node that emitted a light electrical pulse when approached too closely. As the fish swam around peacefully, Sage plunged a plastic shark into the water, scaring little crap strings out of the guppies and causing them to scatter. He had a number of lasers spanning the tank that recorded how many fish swam toward the pellets, a salve of sorts to ease their pain, or toward the unpleasant electrocuting strobe light. Invariably, significantly more fish swam toward the strobe, confirming Sage's theory that guppies, and therefore people, are trauma addicts. He received an honorable mention rather than a ribbon due to the fact that his father, a behavioral physicist, or something, at Lawrence Berkeley National Lab, had played more than a marginal role in his son's project.

At age twelve I found this experiment implausible and dismissed it entirely. Were I sitting in the yard, enjoying the sun, and a rabid wolf suddenly lunged at me from the hedge, I'd hardly think, "This is horrible! I'll go get some toaster strudel and then I'll feel better." Nor would I, while being charged by said rabid wolf, start looking for a stack of paper so I could inflict paper cuts. I'd simply flee and hope not to run into the rest of the pack. Initial implausibility aside, I spent the next twenty years characterizing people into Sage's two categories: eaters and strobes.

Andrea, newly resurfaced-Rob-Lowe-autograph-sharing and foot-peeling friend, was the first person I definitively categorized as a strobe. It was a distinction made crystal clear by her behavior at camp the summer between sixth and seventh grades. We were assigned to a cabin with two other girls and a hierarchy immediately developed. Dana was the definite leader, a bossy fourteen-year-old bull dyke about a foot taller than the rest of us and outweighing me by at least forty pounds. She was fair but merciless, authoritative, demanding, unyielding, and hysterically funny, which is why we tolerated her despotism. Noni and I fell comfortably in the middle of this pecking chain. We hid our fear of Dana and she usually treated us respectfully.

Andrea, however, masked no emotions and dragged miserably from the bottom. She was quiet and submissive, often openly fearful in Dana's presence. She cowered when Dana roared, demanding that Andrea take her funky-ass, corn chip–reeking shoes outside and wash her goddamned putrid feet before she got beat with a lanyard. Andrea would slink out and scrub her moist little toes under the hand pump. Then she'd sulk until one of our counselors—the pot-smoking ball flasher, the stripper, or the one recovering from a recent abortion—banished her to their customary punishment: hugging a massive redwood tree until they remembered she'd been sent away.

This particular morning we four adolescent girls sat in the camp washhouse. It was a primitive structure with a dirt floor and ceramic sinks with built-in washboards. They were practically smooth from years of usage and relatively useless for the purpose of cleaning clothes. We rubbed and scrubbed but the dirt clung to the fabric. Dana had spent about an hour cleaning her lesbian-style painter paints. Her hands were raw from scrubbing and wringing the heavy denim. The pants were still dripping wet when she handed them to Andrea to hold while she prepared to hang them. Andrea foolishly took this opportunity to drop Dana's jeans onto the dirt floor.

It was as though my friend had been suddenly transformed into a jack-in-the-box. Her head bobbled and she looked at Dana with a vapid, drooly grin that Dana immediately wiped off her face by picking up her filthy jeans and slapping Andrea with the not insignificant amount of wet canvas. She then dumped the jeans back into the sink and resumed her scrubbing.

Nobody said a word. The slap echoed in the tin shed. Andrea's face dripped muddy water and a purple welt surfaced on her cheek. Suddenly, a great howl rose up from her core.

She spun on her heels and ran out of the building. I came to my senses and rushed out after her but only caught a brief glimpse of her disappearing into the woods, still howling and hunched over like a feral orphan.

At the time I couldn't understand why Andrea let the pants fall from her grip. Surely she must have known it would lead to a savage beating? It wasn't until the following spring, at the science fair, that I learned she was a strobe. She embraced her suffering.

But fundamentally, Sage's experiment was flawed. His basic assumption was that guppies and people make choices. He didn't take into account all of the fish that were pushed toward the food by the water displaced by the shark. How many of the fish saw the shark as an event, not an opportunity?

Cancer was my shark. Sure I went to treatment and made the small decisions associated with that, but really nothing about me had changed: not my perspective, my goals, nothing. I just floated through life, all pointless and quirky, thinking, "This is so entertaining. I'm so pleased with myself." I spent months upon months actively wondering when I would really realize, like Thibault already had, that everything I was putting myself and my family through could be more than an event.

When I left for college my father gave me a plaque. Plaques of *New Yorker* cartoons and allusive quotations lined his den walls: over the bookcase, "Never read a book, Johnny, and you'll be a rich man"; over his desk, a cartoon of a jungle woman chastising her husband with the caption, "Stop saying it's a jungle out there and get to work!" The plaque he gave me read: "There are no miracles, there is only discipline."

I carried that thing, and it was five by ten inches and a good inch thick of laminated Masonite, to every office or workspace in every town and country I ever lived. And while I had no room for athlete's foot powder while I hiked through the Guatemalan jungle in perpetually wet, leather boots, down in the bottom of my backpack was the plaque. And now, not only was it nowhere to be found, but I found myself actually waiting for a miracle. Not the miracle to save my life, but the miracle to make something of it.

chapter twenty-seven

I had just spent thirty minutes cleaning the bathroom at a Subway restaurant, not because I worked there, but because Lucas, almost two and a half years old, had made *la diarrhée* in his training underpants. I'd almost gotten his pants off without the soupy mess smearing on his legs when he freaked out and started kicking. Poop—baby shit is called poop, but still smells like shit—flew all over the room, splattering the walls and every other surface, including me. Lucas was screaming and jumping into my arms. Some asshole was knocking at the door. I had to give the baby a full bath in the sink, wash off myself and my clothes, and disinfect the entire bathroom with wipes and hand sanitizer, which is more than most people would have done. Most people would have cleaned off themselves and left the bathroom filthy and shit-splattered for some poor illegal alien to clean later. Once it was clean, I sat down to pee and discovered two things: a blob of shit on my big toe and the reappearance of It.

I was either Stephen King's Carrie or a character in a Judy Blume novel, but whichever one, she thought she was dying for about thirty seconds, which is a long time to think you're bleeding to death in front of your child in a public restroom. Then I realized I'd been reinitiated and screamed really, really loudly. It would have scared the shit out of Lucas had there been any left in him.

Thus began my second adolescence or whatever they call that wretched hormonal stage when newly menstruating females are so filled with toxic negativity there is no place for demons like them outside of Hell. I looked at the people who loved me and had cared for me and I wanted to scratch at their faces with rusty barbed wire. There was no sign of the gratitude I should have felt even having PMS or any normal reproductive behavior after chemotherapy.

Dr. Stone called my ovaries "hard core." Less than 4 percent of women resume ovulation after chemotherapy. He was impressed that they'd bounced back, but not happy. He warned me not to get pregnant. It was irresponsible, he said. I had to think about that. The last person who'd called me irresponsible was an administrator at the school where I taught, Josefina-Maria Cagampang. She was a strange person, a skinny little Filipina skeleton with a hairpiece the kids joked she washed in the dishwasher, and a hairy mole on her cheek. She was slightly hunchbacked and had bulging eyes that rolled constantly but never blinked. She chain-smoked and drove her Trans Am with the windows sealed shut and clouds of smoke swirling inside. The first time I "met" her, she marched into my classroom, completely unannounced, without acknowledging me in any way, and started ranting at my students.

"You wanna mess with me? I don't think so. I'm the littlest vice principal you'll see but I got big attitude and the big guns to back it up! You can call me Ms. Cagampang, or Ms. C. Any questions?" Nobody said anything. "You better have something to ask me!" One brave boy raised his hand. "Don't raise your hand while I'm talking!" The classroom was a sea of big round eyes. Then someone paged her on her walkie-talkie and she marched back out of the room taking huge pimplike strides. The kids looked at me. All I could say was that she was clearly insane and if they had any sense at all they'd avoid her at all costs.

One of my students was an angelic-looking, extremely disturbed boy who drew violent cartoons on his desk and scratched himself until he bled. He was the sort of child my mother had in mind when she said abortion should be legal until the fetus is eighteen years old. This day he was stabbing at the kids around him with a compass, one of those V-shaped metal things that has a pointy end and an end that holds a pencil. Not only was he disturbing the other students, but he really could have hurt them. So I sent him to the office. Five minutes later he reappeared at my door.

"Ms. C. told me to come back."

"Go back to the office."

Five minutes later he reappeared.

"Ms. Cagampang told me to come back." This time he said it in robot voice.

"What? No, go back to the office. Tell her I'll come after class."

Five minutes later he was back at my door. This time I wrote a note explaining exactly what he'd done and sent him back to the office.

"Ms. C. told me to come back," he said, his eyes rolling all the way back into his head.

I sent him out and locked the door. Since I was in a portable on the periphery of the campus, my door was the only one that could be locked from the inside and not unlocked from the outside. It was some sort of safety measure. I explained to the kids that if Ms. Crazy-Ass Josefina-Maria Cagampang came to the door, we were to ignore her. Nobody was to laugh or make any sound. We'd pretend like we just didn't hear her.

Five minutes later she tried to open the door. I could see her through the little window searching the room frantically with her bulbous eyes. Then she started knocking. When I didn't open the door she started banging and yelling at me, threatening to call the fire department. After several minutes she disappeared.

After class, when I went to confront her in her office, she said two incredible things: one was, "So, where are these alleged stab wounds?" as if I should have waited until he succeeded in drawing blood before removing him; and two was, "Irresponsible people like you are the enemy of the state."

I called her an idiot and she spent the next two years doing everything she could to get me fired. But of all the names she called me during the time we worked together—*antivisionary, tardy-kin* (which I assumed meant late all the time, not family of retarded people, both of which I was)—the only one that made any impression was *irresponsible*. And now, for the second time, someone was using that same word and again I was baffled. Maybe I didn't know what it meant?

Perhaps my eggs were damaged and the baby would be deformed? Perhaps my body was too fragile and another pregnancy would add undue stress? Perhaps Dr. Stone thought there were already too many babies in the world?

"No," he explained, "the cancer could reappear any time and you wouldn't want to leave *two* orphans."

When he wasn't being a jerk Dr. Stone was a funny guy, handsome and fit. He looked like a runner but swore he didn't run. He didn't seem to approve of running, saying, "True, runners live longer, but they spend all that time running. Or maybe they don't live longer, it just seems longer." He used to hug me hello. Dr. Stone was very sweet; he seemed fond of me and I never felt Frewed.

Finneas Frew was a man I worked with in New York. He assaulted everybody he knew, male or female, with these really intense, lingering hugs or viselike handshakes where, after the appropriate three shakes, he refused to let go of your hand and would instead swing it playfully until you peeled his fingers off yours. I got to be so terrified of his unsolicited embraces that I rearranged the furniture in my office, making it impossible to touch me without climbing over a credenza. When Finn was around I never left my desk without one of those big boxes of paper reams. It was empty, but I pretended it was really heavy and awkward to carry. It blocked the hug attempts, as even Finny Frew wasn't weird enough to hug me from behind, and kept my hands convincingly unavailable for shakes.

A few weeks into extended therapy I brought Thibault to an appointment and upon seeing him Dr. Stone stopped dead in his tracks. "Who is this?" as if I held the man next to me on a leash.

"My husband?"

Dr. Stone turned around and left huffily.

"Are you having a love story with your doctor?" Thibault asked.

"Not that I know of," I said, secretly pleased.

When Dr. Stone returned a few moments later he introduce himself to Thibault and shook his hand. "You must be the husband." Then he proceeded with the examination. The next time I came alone. Dr. Stone said, "So, is he rich, you know, of means?" as if Thibault weren't a total fox, like he needed to be rich to get a woman.

"Very," I said, and wondered if they sold organic milk at the Chevron food mart, my gas card being the only credit card not yet maxed.

At my next appointment I asked Dr. Stone about getting breast reconstruction. He'd just given me a breast (singular) exam and I sat in front of him topless.

"I was thinking about getting a new one, and the old one fixed up. I wouldn't want a new saggy one to match the old saggy one; and I sure don't want a perky new one to mismatch the old saggy one."

"What are you talking about?" he asked.

"The old boob is not cute. I want two cute boobs."

He studied it indifferently. "It looks cute."

But he only said it to be polite. Without my shirt there was none of that flirtation I was used to in his voice. It was a combination of professionalism and utter lack of sexual interest.

When did men start looking at my tits and stop getting hard-ons? I hoped when it went from tits to tit. But in reality, it happened before that, when I stopped being young enough to be a young mistress. It had already started the day I caught that overtanned, Rolex-wearing tool check me out, shrug, and just as quickly dismiss me, thinking, clear as day, "Puh, I could do better." I laughed out loud it was so insulting.

But then I got pregnant, which meant I wasn't totally undesirable, gained all that weight, went bald, and had a mastectomy. The flirtation with Dr. Stone had been potentially inappropriate, but harmless, welcome, and a sweet little reprieve. I liked feeling beddable again, even if nobody had any intention of acting on it. What was ahead for me: the required affection of my husband and, at best, kind and platonic smiles from other men? Things could definitely be worse, but it still just sucked.

Every day I was less and less of the taut brown girl on the dressing bench in the YMCA, the girl sitting amid all the damp bathing suits surrounded by the crepey, sagging, wrinkled skin, bowed spines, and liver spots of the naked old ladies fresh out of the steam room. I used to sit there after my swim lessons, gawking, eyes darting about, biting my nubby fingernails with my giant incisors until my sister, at my mother's insistence, came and found me.

I thought that my body would never look like theirs. It would never bend and shrink. Sure I'd die and have a funeral, but I'd be there watching, sitting in the back in my roller skates, the same ones I wore to bed. I never imagined myself still and lifeless, with just a touch of lip gloss, like a polished seashell. I never imagined myself with one saggy, not cute breast and scars all over, half-blind and half-witted from the chemo.

I used to think about how my life would be different after "the Event" that kills off most of humanity but leaves me and a few others unscathed. We would be left to fend for ourselves. (I always thought the first thing I'd do is run to Costco and get a lifetime supply of toothbrushes.) But since starting the second round of chemotherapy, I'd been considering what would happen if I did not survive, what would happen to my body with nobody left to dispose of it properly, to clean it, dress it up, and pose it in a comfy carved box, like they'd done for my grandmother and, more recently, for our family friend Lawrence.

Lawrence's funeral was the first I'd been to in at least ten years, and certainly the only one I'd been to since getting diagnosed. When I entered the funeral parlor lobby, a close family friend, currently in chemotherapy, gave me a look that almost made me laugh out loud. It said, "Glad to be a guest. I know *you* know what I mean." I kissed his cheek—smooth from hair loss, not from shaving—and asked him how he felt. "Good!" he piped, as if *good* and *alive* were synonyms. Then I went inside, took a brief look at the body in the open casket, and thought, "Where's Lawrence?" like the real Lawrence would have been standing behind the casket offering me gumbo, not in it looking excessively slack-faced, smileless, less animated even than one of Maple's mice.

Lawrence had lost his battle, but was there any chance, ever, of his winning the war? What did that even mean? You're winning as long as it's not your funeral? Like the War on Drugs and the War on Terror, this war had no clear enemy. Was it the disease or the dying? And if there was no winning, what was the objective? Perhaps just to fight as long as possible with as high a quality of life as possible. I'd captured some ground, reclaimed a fort, whatever lame war metaphor signified getting back my ability to breed, but I still lived in too much fear of insurgency to feel safe enough to use it.

chapter twenty-eight

Treatment finished with very little ceremony. Twenty months after being diagnosed I had my last infusion and Dr. Stone drank a bottle of Martinelli's Sparkling Apple Cider with me. Thibault and I didn't even go out to dinner, which was fine with me; I preferred to celebrate things that were happening versus things that were not.

A few days later I caught Thibault gazing at me with a disheartened frown and I could only guess the source. It might have been the fact that I was eating in bed in my street clothes, or that he blamed me for the disappointing state of our lives. The elation of having survived cancer, and I couldn't really say that we'd done that just yet, but the elation we expected when I stopped treatment with a clean bill of health amounted to nothing more than the disappearance of dread. Reclaiming our future should have made us feel empowered like Lance Armstrong. Instead we felt like any character played by Bill Murray.

I asked him what he was thinking, and after a long silence he said, "Life is often a struggle and it takes away all the peps and the funny times." It would have been really poignant had it not been said with his accent.

Perhaps Thibault just wanted normalcy again, a life where a skin blemish was just a zit and shortness of breath meant I was out of shape, not showing first signs of metastasis. His frowns led me to believe, however, that, like me, he wanted my cancer to wisen us, to bring us some answers to life's key questions, and force our evolution. Instead, there we were, with the same annoying habits and bad manners, ungrateful, pessimistic, undisciplined, and bored. We were just as mediocre as when this whole drama began, even more so, because we'd paid the price for enlightenment.

Early on, a few days after my diagnosis, as I walked across the parking lot toward my borrowed car, I had had a blinding revelation. I actually expected to have many life-altering epiphanies that caused me to motivate or change myself, my family, my country, or the world. I would discover new aptitudes, have an adroitness in areas where competence had always eluded me. It would be either a divine gift or a convenient side effect of my medications, but somehow, I'd jump-start into action.

My father always described me as a successful but poor student. This meant I got good grades but managed to avoid learning anything. This was true in every subject save science, where in high school I excelled. But by college I only took the requirements. I took Physics for Poets, didn't even buy the textbook, and got a 7 percent on the midterm. I pulled myself together, getting an A on the final, but ended up with a C in the class, which I considered a great injustice as the final was cumulative.

I also took Dinosaurs. It was a geology/paleontology class offered for the first time my sophomore year. The big lavender sauropod on the textbook cover was a blatant con. That class required unreasonable amounts of memorization. It was so complicated that people couldn't even formulate questions for the professor. They'd be like, "Did the psaur, brac, ornita, pods, saurs, have ischia, illia, never mind."

That class also marked the most embarrassing moment of my college career. It was indeed more embarrassing than receiving a 7 percent, fourteen out of two hundred points on a Physics for Poets midterm. The professor was talking about teeth and the similarities that linked species and genera, or something. He said that pig and human teeth were so similar that even dentists can't distinguish them; consequently, they are often used when people fake their own deaths. I chose this moment, after ten weeks of inconspicuous silence, to raise my hand and ask the question, "Pigs have teeth?" My friends were mortified. I had, however, performed a great service to the rest of the students. As a result of my question, the bar was lowered to such a subterranean standard that people felt much more comfortable asking basic questions. Suddenly, asking if a trilobite was aquatic or if an antorbital fenestra, the hollow cavity behind the eye socket, was part of the sinus system made you look like a genius. At least you knew that pigs had teeth, especially after the professor had just lectured about pig teeth for ten minutes.

Obviously, my scientific prospects were not too promising in college. I abandoned my dreams of orbiting the Earth in the International Space Station for liberal arts studies. I changed my major four times, from religion to art history to English and finally film. It was all a tremendous waste of time and I felt supremely guilty vis-à-vis my father for the years of saving and sacrifice he made to pay my full tuition at a private college.

But despite my poor performance and lack of initiative or natural ability, I still harbored this belief that my great contribution to humanity would be in the field of science. And since the early days of my cancer treatment I hoped I'd wake up one morning with a photographic memory and genius math skills, skills that would bring clarity to a vision I'd had since I was small.

The vision was of the edge of the universe. There is much debate and speculation as to this mysterious zone. If the universe is expanding, what is it expanding into? Nothing is not empty space, but the absence of space. Assuming the big bang theory is true, the entire universe began as one single point of energy. It was not a point of energy suspended in a vacuum of empty space, but a point that encompassed all space. For someone inside this point, there would be no outside. Nor could anybody be outside to view what this point of energy even looked like.

The big bang expanded into what? At ten years old I perfectly understood that it expanded into itself. There was no such thing as a straight line; space was curved. Each side of this point of light expanded in a curved line into its opposite side, thus creating a crazy doughnut shape with the hole obscured by the doughnut itself. If you traveled far enough from the center of the doughnut, you'd find yourself pushing against a rubbery wall of plasma. On the other side of that wall would be the opposite edge of the universe, 180 degrees behind you and equidistant from the core of the explosion.

As the universe expands, actual space is created between these rubbery fields of plasma. The reason the expansion is accelerating is because as space is created between these walls, it forms a vacuum that sucks the existing universe into it. It provides a force of acceleration.

All I needed, to become more famous than Albert Einstein or this year's American Idol, was the mathematical proof. Unfortunately, I didn't even know what that meant. I had no idea how to formulate an equation or a proof as any type of support. I didn't even know what the variables would represent.

At my college graduation the school conferred several honorary degrees. One was to Gertrude Elion, who had won the Nobel Prize for designing powerful drugs to combat childhood leukemia. She also created drugs to facilitate organ transplants and for treating herpes. People could hardly keep their eyes open during her acceptance speech. They were audibly yawning and tossing around a beach ball. She received lukewarm applause at the end.

The other honorary degree went to Katharine Hepburn. She blew sunshine up her own ass for half an hour while the audience sat enraptured. They burst into applause and actually gave her a standing ovation at the end. What had she contributed to society? What dying children had she saved from sexually transmitted disease? I was appalled and defiantly interrupted my fervent clapping to scream "Bravo!"

If I could find the Unifying Theory, the answer to my universal equation, I'd have the acclaim due Dr. Elion, but awarded to Katharine Stupid Hepburn. I'd win the Nobel Prize and parents could facetiously start calling their pubescent boys "Real Meredith Nortons."

And even after teaching, when I went back to study engineering and really put my heart into it, made a real effort by doing all the reading, going to lectures, going to office hours, and hiring tutors, it was clear that any contributions I made to math or physics would be unintentional. I might stumble across some great discovery while searching for something else, but frankly, they told me, I was more likely to grow a tail. (Although now, after all the radiation I've had, that remark is less insulting.) With enough effort I could trudge through and eventually graduate, but I certainly wouldn't be a superstar prodigy publishing in journal after journal and filling big lecture halls. It would take a miracle.

Cancer was the miracle, the catalyst that would pull me out of mediocrity and into distinction. It would at least motivate Thibault and me to improve ourselves in some way, to read rather than watch television, to eat together as a family more often, something. But the way Thibault looked at me showed that in his eyes I was the same sort of cancer survivor as I had been a student, successful but poor, meaning I lived, but managed to learn nothing. Coming out of treatment, my family was nothing more than two years behind schedule. My parking lot epiphany two years earlier was that there might be no lesson in this experience; it might just suck. Thibault had reached the same conclusion. His disappointment was tangible.

The question became what to do with myself now that life no longer revolved around avoiding death. I was thirty-five, no spring chicken, but not exactly a salmon swimming upstream either. I decided to join the rest of America and work on getting out of debt.

Aside from my three-month checkups and the absurdly

lingering effects of colds due to my weakened immune system, I was as close to normal as I had ever been. I wrote, took Lucas to school, and nagged my husband like a good wife. Months passed without event.

Then I started noticing my arms falling asleep, tingling in my fingertips, and pain in my ribs. My arms were either throbbing or like two slabs of meat hanging from my shoulders. Dr. Stone said perhaps I had an "impinged" nerve and ordered spine X-rays. That kept me calm for three days and then I Googled my symptoms and found that they implied spinal or bone cancer, two of the more likely metastasis of inflammatory breast cancer.

Numbness spread to my brain. This time it would be worse. Spines and bones are fairly necessary body parts. Since my arms were exhibiting the symptoms, the affected area would have to be high, near my neck. Hence the neck X-rays. That could mean paralysis, quadriplegia, a motorized wheelchair. If I did end up in a wheelchair I wasn't buying any goddamned minivan to drive around in. Thibault would have to fold my limp ass into a Saab 9-3.

My potential spinal cancer and the impending need for a minivan was not information Thibault needed. I would wait for my test results and then share the doom with my husband. That left five days of personal, internalized hysteria, which I vented occasionally by repeatedly, violently ramming the shopping cart into the metal railing of the Safeway parking lot shopping cart corral, or by throwing handfuls of gravel at the wild turkeys shitting on my driveway. I never misbehaved with a human audience, so my dread went unnoticed.

The night before my appointment I felt a sore on my back, close to the spine about waist level. Not being able to see it clearly, due to its inconvenient location, I had to let Thibault look. He said it was red and swollen, but more blistered than infected-looking. I was sure the new spine cancer had spread to my skin, just as it had on my breast. Again, I said nothing. Thibault just shrugged and told me to let Dr. Stone see it in the morning.

Thibault insisted that I listen to this French radio podcast during my half-hour drive to the medical center. He loaded it on my iPod and had it waiting for me in the car when I left for my appointment. As I drove down my familiar stretch of highway the hosts talked about soccer (boring) and Lance Armstrong again (more boring). What else could they possibly say about doping? Jesus and Mary, the French were determined to find some drugs in that man's system. I was tempted to turn it off and already thinking of what to say to Thibault for making me listen to that crap when I heard the thing that made me ashamed of ever doubting my husband. When asked about the French 2006 FIFA World Cup team, Lance Armstrong was quoted as saying, "All their players tested positive . . . for being assholes." Now he was officially my hero. I'd dig up that yellow bracelet and wear it out of support for that statement alone.

Dr. Stone came into the exam room with a big smile and reported that my X-rays, MRI, and bone scan were clear. I really must have some pinched nerve or something, but there was no evidence of cancer. Then he began to examine me, listening to my heart, lungs, and feeling down my back.

"Geesh, what's that?"

"I don't know. I found it yesterday. I can't see it, really." He bent down to look more closely.

"Hmmn," he said. "Have you ever had herpes?"

"WHATTTT!!!!????? NO!! WHAT!!! HERPES!!?"

"Okay, okay. Calm down."

"What do you mean, herpes?!"

"Genital? Oral?"

"No, for God's sake, no! You think I have herpes on my back!" I was restraining tears.

"Relax. It's just a question. Relax."

"People get herpes on their backs?! My God!"

"It could happen, but let me see. This actually looks like a bite, maybe a spider bite. Do you have lots of spiders?"

"Spiders? I can deal with spiders or spinal cancer or bone cancer—"

"You don't have spinal cancer, Meredith."

"I can live with cancer, Dr. Stone, having it, not having it, waiting, whatever. But I cannot deal with herpes on my god-damned back!"

He just stared at me.

Nothing else has happened, but it will. As my father says, "None of us gets out of here alive." We are still in Sonoma County; most of our stuff is still in storage in France. And that's fine. I don't need it. Currently, there is no fire to put out, but things aren't static enough to be suspenseful, either. There is none of that quiet waiting for disaster to strike. My life is back to being as normal as it ever was.

We are celebrating Lucas' fourth birthday, a jungle adventure, on the third anniversary of my cancer diagnosis. The statistics suggested I wouldn't live to see my son turn four. I know I should be more actively grateful, maybe volunteer, see Al Gore's movie, send Girl Scout cookies to the soldiers in Iraq, something. Instead, all I can think about is how awesome Lucas' party will be and how I can't wait to have forty people, a serval cat, a ten-foot albino python, and a real, live alligator in my tiny, one-room house. Thank God there are other people to worry about the big stuff.

ACKNOWLEDGMENTS

I'd like to thank all the people who have helped me in so many different ways regarding this book: Karen Alexander, Wah Chen, Rue Harrison, Shirin Malkani, Bob Neer, Andrea Quee-ley, Rebecca Whittaker, and Karla Zens. And for a lifetime of support, I thank my parents, John and Eloise Norton; my grandmother, Alexandria Edwards; my siblings, Angela Norton Tyler and Douglas Norton; and sugar baby, Lucas. Angela, especially, without your daily encouragement and brutal honesty I'd probably be living in an adult detention facility. And to my agent, David Halpern, and editor, David Cashion, I can only express how grateful I am to you both for your faith in me. And a very special thanks to John Bemelmens Marciano, who has shown me what true friendship and generosity of spirit are. Seriously, without you this book really would not have happened. For so many others who I'll kick myself for forget-ting, don't be offended; blame it on the chemo. Ah, chemo! I forgot my doctors! Thank you, thank you, thank you.